A Healing Grove

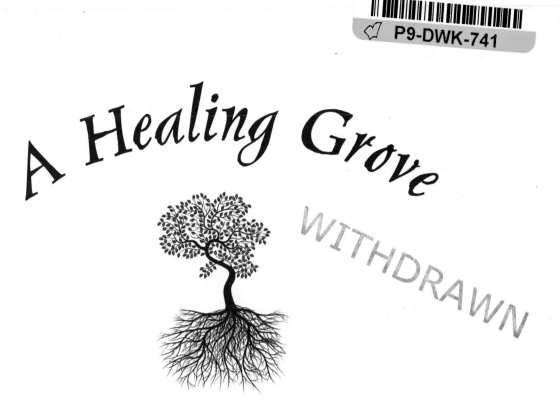

AFRICAN TREE REMEDIES AND RITUALS FOR BODY AND SPIRIT

STEPHANIE ROSE BIRD

Foreword by Judika Illes

Lawrence Hill Books

Library of Congress Cataloging-in-Publication Data

Bird, Stephanie Rose, 1960–
  A healing grove : African tree remedies and rituals for the body and
spirit / Stephanie Rose Bird.
    p. cm.
  Includes bibliographical references and index.
  ISBN 978-1-55652-764-7
  1. African American magic. I. Title.
  BF1622.A34B 568 2009
  615.8'8—dc22
                2008052195

Cover and interior design: Sarah Olson
Illustrations: Stephanie Rose Bird

Published by Lawrence Hill Books
An imprint of Chicago Review Press, Incorporated
814 North Franklin Street
Chicago, Illinois 60610
ISBN 978-1-55652-764-7
Printed in the United States of America
5 4 3 2 1

Contents

This book is dedicated to the oak tree on Spill-way Drive on Paradise Lake that befriended me, the oak that was strong, yet a soft sponge for my tears, a patient caregiver, comfortable seat and support system, and a listener without judgment or opinion, and to my father who kept that tree healthy, strong, and safe in my absence.

A Healing Grove was written with love and gratitude for the lessons learned and those yet to come . . . lessons of the oak.

Acknowledgments

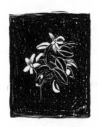

Special thanks to Daniel Zima and Jannette Giles-Hypes for their careful help and attention to detail in the developmental stages of this book. Thanks to Yuval Taylor for believing in this project from early on. Heartfelt thanks to Susan Branadini Betz for kind support and editorial input throughout the project. Thanks also to the editorial, art, and PR teams at Lawrence Hill Books, Independent Publishers Group. Thanks to the creator and the Great Goddess for shepherding this book through its many twists and turns. Blessed Be!

Foreword

JUDIKA ILLES

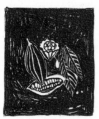

The highest praise that I can give a book is to say that I wish I'd written it; *A Healing Grove: African Tree Remedies and Rituals for the Body and Spirit* is one such book. Stephanie Rose Bird—visual artist, educator, brilliant herbalist, evocative writer—has crafted a crucial and important book, sharing valuable, rare information that has never been more needed and relevant than it is today.

She tells the story of the sacred wood: how to live in it, learn from it, derive spiritual enrichment from it, and how to preserve and protect it. *A Healing Grove* is packed not only with information but also with functional, accessible recipes, remedies, and rituals to serve mind, body, soul, and spirit, derived from a variety of African and African American traditions.

No newcomer to these traditions, Bird's book follows her journey from New Jersey's Pine Barrens (a true seer, Bird is able to recognize the Pine Barrens as a powerful sacred grove) across the United States. Africa is always the touchstone, the persistent and tenacious ancestral mother wisdom and spiritual foundation that refuses to fade away.

Reclaiming botanical and herbal information has never been more important than it is today. So much of our future depends on our ability to reclaim and use ancient Earth knowledge. Although many botanicals and herbals have been published, they tend to focus on Europe and the Americas.

For many, the word *rainforest* is synonymous with the endangered Amazon Basin, as if that were Earth's only endangered patch of healing green. Africa, the Mother Continent and allegedly the birthplace of the entire human race, remains largely ignored. Yet African wild lands are as endangered as the Amazon. Equally endangered are the traditional indigenous cultures of Africa, caretakers of sophisticated botanical medicinal systems whose roots stretch back to the proverbial dawn of time.

A Healing Grove preserves this knowledge, presenting it as relevant and viable and demonstrating in intimate detail how vestiges of that knowledge took root in the Western Hemisphere, in African American culture, and in American culture, period. *A Healing Grove* celebrates the forest: its powers, spirits, magic, medicine, and mysteries.

Bird intimately shares how trees have provided her with personal healing, and then allows us to share in that process for our own benefit and, by extension, provide healing for Earth's beleaguered forests, a potent rehabilitation of centuries of defamation of wild nature that has left Earth in ecological disaster and humans in spiritual distress.

The book is about African tree medicine for a new world, not just the Western Hemisphere but for the entire Earth on the brink of the twenty-first century, the brink of a new age, a new world. We stand at the crossroads between paradise and ecological disaster; *A Healing Grove* points us in the sacred and healthy direction.

Preface

SEEING THE FOREST FOR THE TREES: STORY WITHIN *A HEALING GROVE*

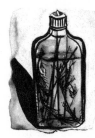 I owe my early camaraderie with the woods to my patience, my willingness to search, and my love of mystery. The trees became my friends after my family moved from an urban suburb near New York to the desolate Pine Barrens of New Jersey. My father's logic for moving from the city to the country seemed counter-intuitive. Most African Americans had begun the sojourn from the South and rural areas to cities in the early decades of the twentieth century, but in the late 1960s we moved to a rural community in the Delaware Valley. Whereas both sets of my ancestors had lived in Virginia, my father's people having lived in the original shires of that state since the mid-1700s, our families left those rural communities to seek opportunities in the North.

Dad turned the clock back and chose to go against the flow. Believe you me, this move was not easy. Mom hated it for quite a while. On the playground my brother and I had a rude awakening, which replayed itself almost daily. We were still the same, yet somehow now belonged to a different category of humans, taunted in a scathing, hurtful tone with unfamiliar words: *nigger this, nigger that, nigger, nigger, nigger.* Stung by my classmates' response to us, at the age of about seven I turned to nature for solace. As sparse as the Pine Barrens were, there were still more trees than there were racists.

I remember practicing my ballet turns outdoors, barefoot, my sole audience the trees. I picked a favorite tree for focus, using it for spotting to perfect my turns, then I'd spend hours climbing and chilling on a very old oak, relishing my new forest environment that, despite the townsfolk, led to my lifetime passions—art, writing, and dancing.

But this love of the woods does not resonate in us all. Some thought I was a bit touched in the head. And some of the folk who visited from our former urban home were afraid for the sun to set on them in the woods. I remember one uncle in particular, Uncle Jimmy. Quick witted and fast talking, he revealed gold fillings as he spoke. Uncle Jimmy was smartly dressed and originally came from coastal North Carolina. He was dead serious about the sun never setting on him in South Jersey . . . dead serious. Why? I didn't get it at first. I later discovered a special street in town called Nigger Lane—a remnant from the past, I prayed—which was purportedly used for lynching. And I had a glimpse of a life that we as black people thought we'd moved well beyond.

I had thought the fears of my uncle and like-minded relatives were just those of the older generation, always an easy out for youth. Now that I've matured, I understand that these were black folk, relatives, whose elders in turn had heard of tree lynchings; some were directly affected. My skin crawled as I heard recently of how entire families had been lynched in rural areas of my current state, Illinois. Those who stood their ground sometimes died violently upon it.

A noose hanging from a tree remains a powerful symbol and continues to be a tool of terror, never completely vanishing from schools and college campuses. The symbol was resurrected in 2008 during the highly publicized controversy around the noose hung on the only shade tree on the grounds of the high school in Jena, Louisiana.

This connection between blacks and trees in the New World is a grim story; it is shameful that slaveholders turned tree-loving people against the woods. But for many, that is just what happened. The city, with its inherent problems, was where my immediate family fled, like many others, and today the synonym—or shall I say code word?—for *black* is *urban*.

Still, plenty of us remained connected to the woods, and we thrived, not only down South but also in countrified pockets on the East Coast, in the Midwest, and elsewhere. I'm sure you have heard the idioms before: "hicks from the sticks," "country bumpkin," meaning people who hail from the forest. People from the Pine Barrens are called Pineys.

I never really felt shame about being associated with the forest; who would? Just as in a fairy tale where the wood holds mystery and magic that takes place nowhere else on earth, so too are the forest and my story of it—indeed, it is *our* story—a largely untold story of the sacred wood: how to live in it, learn from it, and utilize its precious healing gifts. This is a story that, for our people, has remained silent far too long.

Ase: From the Crossroads!
Stephanie Rose Bird, 2008

Introduction

HOLLY, OAK, AND PINE: ENTER MY PERSONAL FOREST

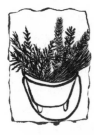 Billie Holiday sang the bittersweet song to perfection, written by Abel Mereopol, a Jewish English teacher and political activist from the Bronx. This song, which *Time* magazine named "Song of the Century," is an ode to lynched African Americans, casting a glaring spotlight on injustice and illuminating some of our uneasiness toward the woods. Rich in the metaphor of a brutal reality, "Strange Fruit" likens the swinging, dull, lifeless bodies of our people to a strange fruit.

Who can fault an African American of the older generation for being afraid of the wood? This fear is a source of some of our country blues, and I don't mean that in a musical way; rather, it is a malaise we feel in colonized lands that was not present in the same way in the Motherland. Yes, we feared animals, reptiles, poisonous insects, some wild spirits, and foreign warriors' clans, but not fellow Americans who would kill us, sometimes simply because of the color of our skin.

I am, however, undeterred, and we as a people have always been that way. The African American spirit of survival has always been strong. While some make their way in the urban jungle, my grounding and centering remains in the forest, as lush and mysterious as it is forgiving yet foreboding. I'm hoping my story of *A Healing Grove* transports you back and forth across the Atlantic on a journey that builds an understanding of the potent healing power of trees, not just for African-descended people but indeed for all, wherever they are rooted.

Trees of Life

When my citified relatives (as we thought of them) came and went from our home during summers and on weekends of barbecuing chicken, ribs, and freshwater fish like largemouth bass, pike, sunfish, and pickerel caught by my dad, they took off from our humble dirt road to asphalt, from three swamp oaks at the beginning of our property. Wacky and weird as those trees were, they are still the emblem of home emblazoned in my mind's eye. To this day, that trio of oaks bears the marks of my siblings and me as we played games growing up, numerous dog and cat scratches here and there, dings from cars and pickup trucks coming a little too close to the trees in their hurry to return to the bright lights of the big city and the lure of towns nearby. For me, oak became and remains the tree of life.

A SINGLE MAJESTIC TREE: SALEM OAK

For African people, trees served as visual markers and potential medicine (such as slippery elm or pau d'arco, as you'll soon see), as well as shade for cooling, with breezes from the leaves welcome. Trees are my way of knowing: where I am, where I am going, where I have been personally and historically.

When I was growing up in Salem County, one of the annual field trips during grade school was to see our old oak tree, with its ever-widening girth, to hear tales of how it began its life over four hundred years ago. Salem County is rich in history as one of the oldest counties of the original thirteen colonies; it was established in 1694. The tree is believed to be the place where John Fenwick signed a treaty with a local native group, the Lenni Lenape, to purchase the land. Since 1681, the Religious Society of Friends (an offshoot of the Quakers) has owned and maintained the land where the oak tree grows. It has been a Friends burial ground for hundreds of years. At the seat of the county, the Salem Oak Tree remains an anchor to major towns of the area; people die, stores and factories close, but the tree remains an emblem of continuity in an area seated on the shore of change.

LIVING AMONG THE OAKS

I have trees and nature within both my name and the map to my self. My middle name is Rose, after my godmother whose strength and beauty aligns her well with that flower; my maiden name, Hunt, and married name, Bird, are also evocative of the natural environment. Though Hunt is not suggestive of woods by itself, it is a shortened, more contemporary name taken by my great-grandfather when he moved my grandma and her siblings north. Our original name is Hurst, an English topographic name for someone who lived on a wooded hill. The German topographic name is derived from the Middle High German *hurst*, meaning "woodland" or "thicket." The closest ancestral relatives I can find in Portugal are named Da Silva, which is a topographic name for someone who lived by a wood, from the Latin *silva* for "wood."[1] Moreover, another developed town near where I grew up, Woodstown, is where I went to high school and where my parents are buried.

My connections do not end in New Jersey. The state tree of Illinois, where I currently live, is also a very real reminder of home: the oak. It is no mistake that the suburb where I reside has an entire Department of Forestry to manage the trees of its thriving urban forest, a village repeatedly noted by the National Arboretum Society as one of our country's top tree towns. The urban forest of Oak Park has Forest Park and River Forest nearby; where else could I set up my house and raise my family? Outside my home grows an oak that is weird, wacky, and wonderfully twisted. That oak tree lets me know the time of day by the shadows it casts, the season by how it speaks, and the mood of our neighborhood through the akashic energy it emanates.

PILSEN NEIGHBORHOOD IN CHICAGO

For years I internalized all these connections to the wood, but I didn't quite understand the feelings until I moved to a loft in the inner city, in Chicago's Mexican American Pilsen community, where there was barely a tree over five years old—at least not around my block or the ones surrounding it in the 1980s.

As I mentioned earlier, at first my mother wasn't so keen on the whole country experience—that is, until she became involved with gardening. She always seemed to be able to grow tomatoes. She even grew cherry tomatoes in our home during the winter, without special grow lights. She just had a green thumb. Remembering how good those tiny tomatoes made us feel when little else seemed to be growing, in my attempt to set up a new home I tried growing tomatoes

> *Wherever you live, you can still be an African-inspired herbalist.*

on the balcony of our loft. The landlord was cultivating what she thought of as a Bohemian look and was in full support. Tomatoes are a traditional food in South Jersey, so much so that they contribute to its nickname, the Garden State; it is why our county hosted Hunt's and Heinz for many years. There is even an oversized, juicy type called Jersey Tomatoes, and, as Aunt Eddie demonstrated on her back stoop, you just had to add a dash of salt and sometimes a bit of mayonnaise and you had yourself some good eating.

But these stock products of home would not grow on that Chicago balcony. I literally thought I would die along with my tomato plants. Not only would my plants not grow on the fire escape, but just exactly how would I know when it was winter, when spring was just about to return, or even when the sun was about to set, without trees?

Eventually, after trying out several types of plants including several temperamental Nordic pines, I reached out to ficus; with the right temperature and a bit of sun, ficus grows anywhere, even inside a loft in Pilsen.

Notes to the Urban Herbalist

A recurring theme in this book is the acknowledgment of urban herbalists. I have lived in very rural environments, suburbs, and various cities. Wherever you live, you can still be an African-inspired herbalist. I give notes and specialized advice to remind you of that ability.

Holly (Ilex spp): Tree of Memory

Typically, a trip home fixed my major tree and plant jones, wherever I lived; admittedly that jones grew out of bounds when I moved to the desert-type terrain of California. Having heard that southern California was so beautiful, my mouth watered as I made my way cross-country, headed to graduate school in La Jolla. Once the plane landed, I realized the sense behind the phrase "beauty is in the eye of the beholder." During my tenure on the West Coast I visited home as many times as possible, even if it was just through my paintings and drawings. La Jolla certainly has it good points; the cove and turquoise-blue sea make it deserving of its name, "The Pearl"; still, its surrounding desert does not warm this heart.

We should never take our indigenous or local trees for granted, because they are precious, as well as being specific markers of home.

The richness of the wetlands and barrens of New Jersey have not only captivated and inspired many an artist and writer, these ecosystems have slowly gained recognition in much wider circles. Eventually, my home on the lake was demolished so that the wetlands could be preserved. The area is earmarked to become a state-preserved conservancy area. Nothing of my physical home is left save memories and all those trees I grew up with, which, with the help of the state of New Jersey, are bound to proliferate.

The last time I visited the area, a magnificent wild holly, about fifteen feet tall with an almost perfectly erect, natural triangular habit, was in full bloom. In the dead of winter this tree greeted me at the bottom of the hill, as I walked back and forth on the dirt road, passing a natural bubbling brook that flows over red earth and pale river rocks, the dam, and the spillway for which the road was named. When I returned home years later, that precious holly was still there and decked in the finery that only rich red berries can offer. Tears streamed down, nestling in the fibers of my down jacket, and they threaten to do the same now as I remember how branches of holly were annually cut by Dad and carted inside to decorate for the Christmas season.

Holly's deep green, leathery leaves and vibrant red berries brightened many a holiday spirit, no matter what else we had or didn't have. The bittersweet joy holly brought that day was short-lived. I was on the way to Salem Hospital to visit my father; he was hooked up to machines and not expected to live long, because that unnatural state was against his living will.

I write about holly in past tense because for a good while it was a part of my past. Holly grows readily in southern New Jersey, but not so well in the Midwest's harsher winter climate. Those boughs and wreaths created lovingly by my parents from Jersey holly became a luxury I could no longer afford, living where I do; one would have to fork over big bucks to a company like Smith and Hawken, or special order from a local florist, for what would still only be a temporary pleasure. This goes to show one of the major lessons of this book: we should never take our indigenous or local trees for granted, because they are precious as well as being specific markers of home.

While not useful for the cancer and pneumonia that besieged my father's lungs, holly has numerous recorded uses among early African Americans along the southeast coast, particularly in Gullah medicine. Holly's leaves were boiled with pine tar, strained, and served warm as a drink to bring down fever. Holly leaf tea was also used to hasten recovery from measles.[2]

I returned after my heartbreaking visit home and found, much to my surprise, a holly sapling, which I did not plant, growing beneath my peony bush just as spring finally appeared. While I thought I was all cried out, that sweet little emblem of home brought more stinging tears to my eyes. It was almost as though it was planted by memory and yearning concerned with place, or stranger still, my father's spirit since he had passed on. This new seedling grew from memories of home, and to this day I tend it carefully. Due to our harsh winters, until it grows too large I'll let it grow strong shielded by the peony, spirituality, and faith.

Pine: Rooting the Ancestors to Community

Historically, trees have been markers for our people. In the early days of life in the Americas, people of African descent wanted trees planted on their burial sites.[3] The tree was usually a conifer, what we call evergreen, as it serves as a reminder of the persistence of life. The trunk, branches, and leaves exist in the realm humans see, while the life force of the tree, the roots, lay beneath the earth. Evergreens are a metaphor for the interaction between departed spirits and their living community.

Elsewhere in the African diaspora, the symbolic tree that serves a similar purpose is the silk cottonwood, which will be explored later.

According to Robert Farris Thompson in *Flash of the Spirit*, pine (*Pinus spp.*) and spruce (*P. Picea*) trees in particular play a key role in traditional Southern U.S. burials, owing to their availability in the region.[4] To early black Americans, the green scent of evergreen trees contained healing medicine for mind, body, and spirit. Dr. Faith Mitchell lists a variety of conditions pine was used to treat in her book *Hoodoo Medicine*: stuffy nose, fever, stomachache, whooping cough, bacteria, parasites, and fatigue. The indigenous people of the Southeast coast used pine tar for swelling, burns, itching, sore throat, colds, and consumption; these applications influenced African American healers as well.[5]

A highly touted organization that quantifies and measures the chemical constituents and efficacy of herbal remedies, the German Commission E (Expanded Edition), states that, while various pines have been used medicinally, including shoots of black spruce, dwarf pine, and longleaf pine, medicinal pine needle oil is derived from steam-distilled essential oil of *Pinus silvestris* L., taken from fresh needles, branch tips, or a combination. The commission approves the use of pine needle oil internally for lung ailments and externally for rheumatic and neuralgic ailments. Pine oil is also used as a fragrance in cough and cold remedies. Those with bronchial asthma or whooping cough are advised against using it. Pine can cause irritation of the skin or mucous membranes, so testing and observation periods are important before using it therapeutically. The council recommends using conifer essential oils in aromatherapy by adding several drops of the oil to hot water and inhaling.[6] Pine is available as a prepared product, and it is also included in various soaps (pine tar), shampoos, conditioners, baths and salt soaks, and ointment rubs.

My grandfather, who was born on a plantation in Virginia in the late 1800s, used tiny portions of oil of turpentine, a by-product of pine, as an antiseptic. In fact, he swore by the stuff, claiming it could make just about anything feel better, from a cut to the common cold. Grand Pop, as we fondly called him, came to live with us in the Pine Barrens, a place so named because it contains so many stands of pine forest. The entire lower half of New Jersey is designated as a pine plain, and conifers grow readily there. Alloway, the tiny town where Grand Pop came to live with us until his death, is one of the isolated outer areas of the Pine Barrens.

In Alloway, pine was all around, and thankfully it remains so. On our drives to the shore you could see sparse forests of pine. Sometimes they had succumbed to spontaneous fire; burnt wood springing from marshes and swamplands lends an eerie quality, reminding us that pine is most definitely a tree of the spirit realm.

Directly outdoors behind our home was a sparse forest dominated by pines and oaks. The one across the lake was a completely different biome: a lush wetland wood. Knotty pine was used as a wall covering in the log cabin we first stayed in, and for firewood to heat the cabin and to heat our bath water, and during holidays pine decorated our living environment.

In case you make it down to that area, the main trees of the Barrens are

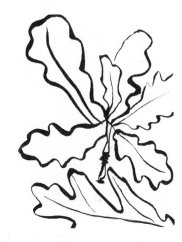

- ≫ Shortleaf pine (*Pinus echinata*)
- ≫ Virginia pine (*P. virginiana*)
- ≫ Red cedar (*Juniperus virginia*)
- ≫ Black oak (*Quercus veluntina*)
- ≫ White oak (*Q. alba*)
- ≫ Chestnut oak (*Q. prinus*)
- ≫ Post oak (*Q. stellata*)
- ≫ Blackjack oak (*Q. marilandica*)
- ≫ Scarlet oak (*Q. coccinea*)
- ≫ Southern red oak (*Q. falcata*)[7]

WORKIN' THE PINE

When my mother was nesting, preparing for my youngest sister, the baby of our family, she used pine floor wash to prepare. Pine floor wash contains some antibacterial agents and makes the home feel energized and fresh. Pine cleansing is a tradition I continued with the births of my children, and I still do it whenever there is a stale feeling in the air.

Many African Americans and Latinas grew up with the smell of fresh pine-scrubbed floors, tiles, and bathrooms. Some now reach out for commercial products, but you can easily prepare your own pine-scented products.

When I am cooped up indoors in winter, my spirits grieve the lively spirit of autumn. My homemade pine floor wash has a remarkable emotional influence. These floor washes are recommended as winter tonic for grief, mild depression, and fatigue. Two updated formulas feature essential oils that are antibiotic, antiseptic, and antifungal.

Forever Green Floor Wash

Clip and fill a stockpot three-quarters full of pliable shoots from spruce and pine trees. Add water to cover. Bring to a boil. Reduce to medium-low. Cover. Decoct 25 minutes. Cool. Strain the liquid and drop in essential oils: ½ teaspoon of Scotch pine (*Pinus sylvestris*), and ¼ teaspoon lime (*Citrus aurantifolia*), ¼ tea-spoon black spruce (*Picea mariana*). Stir in 3 tablespoons liquid castile soap with a large stainless steel spoon. Pour the wash into a large bucket. Sprinkle Forever Green Floor Wash on a broom. Sweep and remove debris. Dip a mop into bucket of pine floor wash to cleanse your home environment physically and spiritually.

PREPARED PRODUCTS

As I said, Grand Pop, born at the turn of the last century, believed in the folk ways of his times and liked turpentine as a cure-all. Today, many African Americans continue to use pine tar for skin and scalp irritation and to stimulate hair growth. I like the scent of pine and use it in aromatherapy. Below are some products that encapsulate these ways of using pine:

≫ Grandpa's pine tar shampoo treats scalp disorders that arise from drying winter winds. Pine soap helps dry, itchy, flaky skin.

≫ Kniepp makes an uplifting pine bath that is useful for replenishing energy. It is designed to help ease depression, and it adds zing to the start of the day.

≫ When using pine medicinally as an oral medicine, use according to your naturopath or herbalist's prescription. If you are making your own decoction, it should be at a ratio of 2 grams pine needle to 150 milliliters water. To make a tincture, use 1.5 (grams/milliliter) to 10 milliliters alcohol solution.

≫ An infusion of pine needles can be taken as tea to help treat cold symptoms, or used as a mouthwash for sore throat and laryngitis.

≫ Pine infusion also makes a fine hair rinse.

≫ Chewing white pine freshens the breath, and the needles contain vitamin C.

Warning: Pine is a known allergen. Wear gloves when handling pine essential oils; test skin for allergic reaction twenty-four hours before use. Pine is not advised for use on sensitive skin. Most people should use pine sparingly; other evergreens might be better tolerated.

Woodsy Essential Oils

Essential oils are the essence of volatile, aromatic oils of trees, plants, flowers, seeds, and pods. While white pine is certainly distinctive, cleansing, and cheap, there are many types of essential oils created from conifers. Here are some of the subtler yet still invigorating conifers oils I use in handmade floor washes, hair care products, and soapmaking. These are especially exquisite additions to Yule or Kwanzaa potpourri blends:

≫ Black spruce—this has a mellow, deep woods scent (multipurpose).

≫ Cedarwood—spiced evergreen, deep and powerful (best in bug-repellant drawer sachets).

≫ Fir needle—fir is somewhat brighter and sharper than pine, but not acrid (good for soap, baths, and potpourri).

≫ Juniper berry—deep fruit scent mixed with evergreen (good in soap, floor washes, potpourri, and other botanical crafts).

≫ Ocean pine—a very mellow, almost sweet pine that is rich enough to resonate, makes a welcome addition to the home (multipurpose).

≫ Scotch pine—a familiar though softer scented pine scent (good for floor washes).

What goes with evergreen essential oils, you may ask? Well, all of this family of essential oils mixes well with pure French lavender. They can be sweetened with the addition of tangerine or lime essential oil, and toned down with a touch of oakmoss, vetiver, or patchouli. To heighten and brighten the wood scents in your homemade blends, use frankincense or lemongrass essential oil. To keep the integrity of the evergreen's outdoorsy scent, use 3 parts conifer essential oil of your choice with 1 part from another essential oil suggested.

Holly, Oak, and Pine: The Flower Essences

Pine, holly, and oak renew and empower us in the woods, in the home, and within the body. They even come in the form of flower essences, which are readymade tinctures. Bach's Flower Essences were developed in the 1930s by Dr. Edward Bach, a British physician, who saw dis-ease as the physical manifestation of unhappiness, fear, and worry. During his research, he developed treatments for various specific emotional states using thirty-eight healing flowers and plants—these are known as Bach's Flower Essences. One of the most common mixtures is Bach's Rescue Remedy.

What I found helpful in these tiny vials, modern-day potions if you will, was a potent way of addressing the emotional and psychological states that form around the grief, loss, and confusion of dealing with relationships. Listed below are three amazing ones.

Using a dropper, take these on a fairly empty stomach, with a clean mouth. You take the number of drops indicated on the label under the tongue—this is called sublingual treatment. The essence is believed to go into the bloodstream faster from beneath the tongue. If you prefer, you can instead add the drops to water and drink it. I recommend taking the essences three to four times per day for best results.

➤ Holly—alleviates pain that arises from negative emotions. Holly fights against the advent of hatred, envy, and jealousy.

➤ Oak—assists the workaholic who works past the point of exhaustion.

➤ Pine—combats the tendency toward guilt, something we all struggle with.

Oak King and Holly King: Re-visioning the Holidaze

Sometimes the Internet can be such a wonderful tool. I recently joined a very large circle of African American women through Yahoo.com who have embraced earth-based spirituality, either Wiccan or as self-described Witches; we are several hundred strong. As I write this book, it is just a few weeks before Yule, and it has been so refreshing to meet all these sisters who also celebrate this ancient holiday, many of them doing as I do and bringing elements of their African culture along with them to the table.

We who celebrate it see Yule as the time of a celestial battle. In our minds' eyes, we are privy to the age-old battle between the Oak King and the Holly King, who some see as different gods and others perceive as twins or two aspects of a single god. The Oak King, also called the Golden King, is the light twin, who rules from midwinter to midsummer. The Holly King (Dark King) rules the mysterious half of the year, from midsummer

CONIFERS IN AFRICAN SPIRITUALITY

The Khemetians of ancient Egypt loved trees. Trees were constantly used in rituals; all statues were fumigated with incense smoke from fragrant tree resins and aromatic leaves. Osiris, an important deity, is thought to be, among other things, a tree spirit. He accepts pinecones as offerings. His spirit resides in sycamore and cedar trees.[8]

to midwinter. Neither rules without a battle for the good graces of the Goddess. The defeated twin lies dormant or dies, and is reborn as a baby, growing six months until the battle at Litha (Summer Solstice) or Yule (Winter Solstice).

OBSERVING YULE

We carry bits and pieces of the celestial battle between the gods into our magickal and mundane lives.

- ≫ Some covens reenact the battle.
- ≫ The Yule log always incorporates some oak as a tribute to Oak King. It is lit ceremoniously, the Light King set ablaze, creating a warming fire fit for celebration.
- ≫ Spiky holly is worn as a crown or made into a wreath, which is symbolic of the continuity of life and of our stories.
- ≫ While others are swept up in the glitz and media blitz of Christmas, we see that the underpinning of Christmas is very pagan.
- ≫ Yule is not complete without Yule log cakes (at least at my neighborhood bakery).
- ≫ An indoor lit evergreen tree reminds us of the goddess St. Lucia.
- ≫ Plenty of holly, the colors gold, green, red, and white, and the foods of our ancestors complete the celebration.

The story of the twin kings is inspirational, and much more sensible than the monstrous manifestation that all my friends and readers know I call the Holidaze.

I am fortunate to be African American and pagan, with a very intriguing blended ancestry. The gift of my ancestors means that I have so much to celebrate and to continue to be thankful for. By staying in touch with the root of the holidays, Yule, Kwanzaa, and, yes, Christmas, I receive light during this time that could otherwise be a chasm of spiritual darkness.

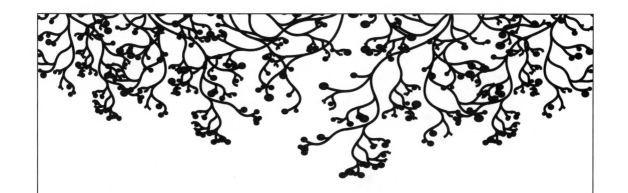

I

Our Heritage and Traditions

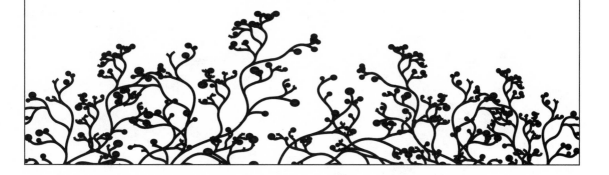

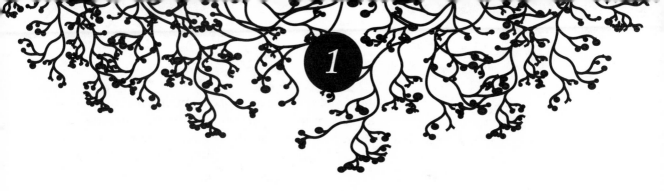

Igboro-Egun

GROVE OF THE ANCESTORS

> *Our ancestors established the sacred groves of Africa and some became African American tree whisperers. Breathless in their wake, we are on a journey of rediscovery, reclaiming Igboro-Egun.*

Celebrating Mystery

Some things are inexplicable. They just *are*. For most, things are explained in various ways: science, faith and belief systems, ancestors, even magick, along with some serendipity. I utilize all of these explanations for occurrences in this book and in my life. I still don't know for sure the real answers, but each of these modes of thinking helps put things into context.

What I did when I found that holly sapling under my peony bush is a good case in point. I did what seems to have come naturally: I thought of its appearance in a mystical way, connecting it to my recently departed father. I promised to shield and nurture it as a symbol of his love and of my childhood home.

Now, as you'll find out in this chapter, various groups of Africans shelter specific trees they deem special. This special tree is called different names by different groups and serves an array of purposes. It may be used to establish and sustain a sense of community, to communicate with ancestors, to connect to deity, or to symbolize place. What I did in my garden was part of a much larger cultural tradition that I did not until recently understand. That is the beauty of being of both Africa and the New World. We are of the oldest people on earth and some of the newest, at once. When those "Africanisms"—habits, customs, or specific types of cultural expressions that are African in origin—pop out, it is wise to take note.

Deep Ancestry: My Inner Forest

As African Americans, we were a disenfranchised group. For many years we felt we would never know where our true homes were—who we are ethnically or tribally, or where exactly we came from. Gradually we came to know through historical accounts that we were most likely sold or stolen from coastal regions of West Africa, what is called the Gold Coast.

Obviously this book speaks about African American people and our relationship to trees. I speak about West Africa often because living there are beautiful, well-defined healing modalities that crystallize the meaning of African holistic health. Moreover, some African American spirituality stems from West Africa's coastal people. During the early drafts of this book I was certain that I was of West African heritage (an educated guess), but I also felt compelled to work in a lot of information about North, South, and East Africa's tree medicines. I didn't know my specific place within it, but I knew that Africa isn't one region but a culturally rich, diverse continent.

But through DNA testing and the study of deep ancestry, I discovered I am not of West African ancestry at all but part of the massive Bantu speakers' migration that led my people south from east Africa—the cradle of civilization. Upon closer investigation, I discovered that my strongest tribal identification is with the Tsongan people, a group from southeastern Africa. I see now why I felt compelled to find out all I could about continental African healing rather than focusing around one area, and I had located my tribal home in one fell swoop.

My test results did shock me, and that is why I took four tests instead of just one. The results are consistent. A consultant pointed me back toward the history of slavery. I took a closer look at statistics and numbers, searching for the truth. It is a historic fact that at least four hundred thousand people of various southern, south-central, eastern, and southeastern tribes were gathered, enslaved, and taken from the shores of Mozambique, near Madagascar.

My secondary ancestry is Mediterranean. It brings in a touch of the Balkans, strongly Portuguese, with a lot of Spanish and Moroccan. There is also just a touch of Albanian/Croatian, and Native American and Oceanic (Aboriginal Australian and western Polynesian) parts are there, but much smaller in comparison. With this discovery I wondered, how could this be? A shout reverberated in my head. Where is the U.S. history to support such ancestry?

As it turns out, Tsongans speak Portuguese as one of their first languages, and it is coming to be understood more widely that the Spanish left their mark in the form of progeny on the southeast coast of the United States, particularly in Virginia (where my people are from) and the Carolinas, but also in Florida and Louisiana, among people who identify as white and black.

Although I felt a connection to Latinos, I was told again and again by the consultant who helped me that the evidence points to Spain, not American Spanish speakers. I would have thought that the Oceanic piece of my ancestry—Australian Aborigine and Western Polynesian—was a genetic impossibility, but it was there as plain as day. I spent time there before I knew, and always felt a connection. Now I have to process what all this means.

My ancestry matches up with African Brazilians because of the Portuguese and African mixture. This book visits with Portuguese-speaking Afro-Brazil to share the benefits of some of the world's superfoods, which grow in the Amazonian rainforest's trees. We stop in to check out the treasures and sustainability projects in East Africa, then to balmy South Africa where just about anything grows, and we sojourn also to West Africa—an important destination if one wishes to learn about African healing ways. I also take you to Australia to glean dreaming wisdom from the black people there who befriended my family.

Showing up with Arab ancestry repeatedly just blew my mind. It didn't match anything I knew, stories or recollections. When I found out it was Moroccan, with my closest affiliation there being the nomadic Berbers, it made more spiritual sense. I understand that the Berbers are so accommodating to foreigners that their phenotype is hard to describe; they are like a rainbow people because they travel and have a history of taking in people, offering refuge. Many of the healing trees that have fascinated me are Moroccan, as you shall see. First of all, though, I want to explore the notion of the grove of the ancestors.

Igboro-Egun: Grove of the Ancestors

I have taken you into my inner forest, even to the deep ancestral level. While the foundations of this book are personal, now is the time to step out of the personal forest together, and go into the deep wood of several African cultures. Learning how to tap into trees to gather spiritual energy is an important legacy of our traditional culture.

Hollywood of earlier eras depicted the African forest as mysterious, dark, and downright dangerous, dubbing it "deepest darkest Africa" and "the jungle." Only the white man Tarzan was capable of maneuvering in such a space and triumphing. What were we in this script? We were "jungle bunnies," of course, which slighted our sexuality, our productivity, and our place of origin all in one ugly idiom. But in our hearts, whether we hail from the city, country, or village, the forest is still fertile, verdant, and in some cases sanctified.

In West Africa, the Yoruba people intentionally create woods, called sacred groves, as places to honor deities and as consecrated grounds, revered by ancestor spirits. These ancestral groves are called *Igboro-Egun*.

Another type of grove, with a different purpose, celebrates specific orisha—the deities of the Yoruba. For example, the *Igboro-Osanyin* is a sacred grove for the orisha of herbalism, the *Osanyin*. *Igboro-Egun* house the *Omiyolo* tree and *Iporogun* and *Atori* shrubs—among the most sacred of trees to the Yoruba.

Many traditional African cultures pay respect to the spirits of trees. There are special dances for specific plants and places, as well as art and crafts to honor nature. Since my childhood, I have done numerous paintings of trees, honoring their presence in my life. The primary focus of my paintings since my earliest years of art school has been capturing the intrinsic spirit of plants and the karma of organic objects.

Other groups of Africans also pay homage to trees and their attendant spirits. Before cutting down a tree, one must address the tree spirits, because evil spirits can also dwell in trees. In *The Healing Drum of Africa,* Yaya Diallo, a master drummer of the Bamana people, tells how a family became mentally ill because they did not adequately follow the protocol for tending to the tree spirits on their land. Purportedly, a tamarind tree next to this family's homestead held spirits that were neither evil nor good. When their father died, the children decided to cut the tree down. Two of the children became disturbed and irrational as soon as the tree was cut. After the spirits lost their tree house they did not want to live alone, so they decided to live within the children and the family on whose property the tree grew. Diallo reports that the family's speech was incomprehensible and says they cried without provocation.[1]

The Bamana people, whom Diallo calls Minianka, live between the Bani and Banifing Rivers in southeastern Mali and northwestern Burkina Faso. Minianka means "those who refuse the master" and refers to the fact that fierce warriors of the area would not relinquish their land or freedom during the French conquest. This group's spirituality is intimately tied to nature. They refused to adopt Islam, a major religion of the area, or Christianity, the minority religion. Demonstrating the importance of the forest to his people, Diallo wrote, "Cultivating a great respect for nature is the ultimate goal of all the customs concerning the sacred wood."[2]

This story makes outsiders privy to a fascinating custom of people of Fienso and Minianka villages, the idea of the first-born tree grove. This small grove, whose center is anchored by a special tree called "first born," is characteristic of villages of Fienso and Minianka people. These groups of people believe that trees and plants have ancestors, just like humans. The first born is the first plant of the creator God, called Kle, and it is the ancestor of all other plants in the area.

Entire groves exist to offer sanctuary to the first-born tree. Only the most esteemed initiates know exactly which plant is the first born, as it is shrouded in secrecy. Most often no one can enter the sacred wood carrying anything harmful to trees such as metal, an ax, or matches.

Some folk believe that evil spirits are sheltered in the wood, so it is unwise to enter without a spiritually grounded guide. Severe punishments are dispensed to anyone who dares disturb the growth or habit of the first-born tree of the sacred grove. If the sacred wood burns, it is considered a very bad omen for the entire community. If such a catastrophe were to occur, a great effort would be made to save the first-born tree so that its role as ancestor to the forest would be preserved, allowing the area to continue to thrive.[3]

Sacred Grove of the Malshegu Community of Ghana

Over centuries, indigenous Africans have lived close to their environment. Their holistic, traditional, and scientific knowledge, which is drawn from experimentation, observation, and innovation, continues to evolve. Taboos, based on spirituality and traditional value systems, have protected biodiversity in Africa. The groves of the Minianka are not singular phenomena. Following is an account of how the Malshegu community of the northern region of Ghana looks upon its wood.

Malshegu is located in the northern administrative region of Ghana, with five thousand people, on the savanna. The settled area came into existence as a way to escape the oppression and rule of Arab invaders from the Sudano-Sahelian region. The Malshegu people are members of the Dagbani ethnic group. Their migration began after the fall of the great empires of ancient Ghana of the twelfth century C.E.

The people have maintained sacred groves, surrounded by Guinea savanna. Women do most of the tending of the crops, as elsewhere in Africa. They use animal manure to ensure soil fertility, and practice crop rotation and intercropping with legumes, allowing six-month fallow periods. The women use hoes and animal traction to prepare the soil. Chemical fertilizers and pesticides are seldom used.

Malshegu people set aside 0.8 hectares of existing open canopy of forest aside for their god, Kpalevorgu. Kpalevorgu takes the form of a boulder under a large baobab tree. The Malshegu believe that the baobab tree helped families over the years, protecting them from invaders. The grove has its own priest, called *Kumbriyili*, who is also the village leader. As the god's sanctuary, this area offers respite from daily goings on, offering peace and quiet. It also provides an overview of the village.

The Malshegu sacred grove is one of few remaining examples of non-riverine, closed-canopy forest in Ghana's savanna. Malshegu sacred grove and god Kpalevorgu's land form part of a rich and complex traditional form of nature conservancy. The grove is a vital habitat, preserving much of the area's fauna and flora and forming a physical focus for Malshegu's spirituality.

The sacred grove is an important location for seeds and seed dispersers, which are vital to local cultivation practices. Home to numerous medicinal herbs, trees, and plants, it has important social and religious functions. A baobab tree anchoring the grove ensures a localized high water table. The forest protects the Malshegu from wind, rain, storms, brushfires, and flooding. According to environmental engineering student Edmund Asare, the sacred grove provides an example of ways that traditional cultures combine religion and cultural practices, leading to successful environmental management, preservation, and sound resource management.[4]

Indigenous–Led Alpine Rainforest Conservancy in Madagascar

While well intended, conservation efforts led by non-indigenous people often fail; as a result, there has been growing attention paid to conservation and sustainability efforts led by indigenous people. Our next segment travels into East Africa, examining the work of an important organization. Seacology, a not-for-profit organization, supports indigenous-led research projects dealing with island ecosystems around the world.

At the time of writing, Seacology was supporting the work of Professor Elisabeth Rabakonandrianina, Ph.D., or Bako as she is affectionately called, who works diligently to protect Mt. Angavokely. Mt. Angavokely is a 1,717-acre oasis of intact, high-altitude rainforest, just fifteen miles outside Antananarivo, the capital city of Madagascar. As it stands, Madagascar is the fourth largest island in the world. Eighty percent of its plant and animal life are endemic (they grow no place else on earth). Madagascar is isolated on the Indian Ocean, 250 miles east of the Mozambique coast. It also has a relationship to African America, since, as I mentioned previously, hundreds of thousands of Africans were enslaved and taken to the New World from Mozambique's shores. Presumably, this is where my ancestors left the Motherland. I have been eager to establish contacts there and to put a face on this mysterious, incredibly large African island blessed with profuse biodiversity.

I had the pleasure of establishing an e-mail relationship with and interviewing Bako, and she is as warm as she is charming. Her passions are recording and preserving the high-altitude rainforest. Her research community is home to more than 120 species of rare and endangered orchids. The forest she studies forms a watershed for three local communities of indigenous people, totaling twenty thousand inhabitants. Seacology and Bako are working with a Malagasy organization called ARVERT, faculty from the University of Antananarivo and Uppsala University, and the Service des Stations Forestieres, to create a new national park at Mt. Angavokely for recreational purposes and research opportunities.[5] Often there are stakeholders from a variety of facilities, making this an optimal way to work.

According to Bako, several medicinal herbs have been found on Mt. Angavokely, including three members of the Asteraceae family:

≫ *Helichrysum gymnocephalum* (DC.) H. Humb—used as an aphrodisiac, antiseptic, and stimulating treatment for bronchitis.

≫ Endemic *Psiadia altissima* (DC.) Benth and Hook—used to make toothpaste and as a treatment for eczema.

≫ Endemic *Bryophyllum proliferum* (Bowie) ex Hook, Crassulaceae—used for coughs.

≫ *Brachylaena ramiflora* (DC.) Humbat, Asteraceae—used to lower malaria fever.

≫ Non-endemics include the fascinating *Siegesbekia orientalis L., Asteraceae*, which is used to stop bleeding and heal wounds. According to Bako, the indigenous name for the plant, *Satrikoazamaratra*, means "I am happy to have wounds because it heals real fast."

The drive to find fuel wood to make good charcoal unfortunately leads to poaching and deforesting. This issue affects just about every indigenous culture and has not left Madagascar unscathed. To prevent massive destruction, Bako developed and introduced an alternative charcoal using forest litter and rice hulls (which are grown locally) instead of hardwood. Bako won the Seacology Prize for her outstanding work in the Manafiafy Forest, a 1,730-acre area composed primarily of one of the last standing littoral forests of Madagascar palm.

Kaya: Sacred Wood of Kenya

A code of behavior emphasizing decorum, respect, and self-restraint protects the ecosystem surrounding the sacred wood.

Along the southern coast of Kenya, sacred forests of the Mijikenda are a long-standing legacy of a people's history, culture, and religion. For centuries, these once-extensive lowland forests have shielded these areas, called *kaya*, meaning homesteads of the Mijikenda; *kaya* shields against invaders while also serving as a space for sacred activity.

As with the Malshegu people of Ghana, and the work of countless groups in all points of the Motherland, social taboos prohibited the felling and removal of trees and other forest vegetation for all but a few purposes, and then only by trusted individuals. *Kaya's* protected status allowed it to become a repository of biodiversity, harboring many rare species of plants and animals. Still, challenges and conflicts between traditional and more Western ideas persist, causing a struggle to preserve the area.

Kaya forest is the domain of nine Mijikenda groups: the Giriaima, Digo, Duruma, Robai, Kauma, Ribe, Jibana, Kambe, and Chonije due to forced migration from southern Somalia. The groups used thick belts of forest as protection. The entire community lived within a single clearing. A protective talisman called *fingo*, representing community identity and history, is buried in a secret spot within *kaya's* clearing. Burial sites located within surrounding forests and shrines honor the graves of great leaders. Social protocols established and enforced by *kaya* elders regulate activities that would otherwise damage *kaya*. Cutting trees, grazing livestock, and collecting or removing forest materials were all strictly forbidden.

Over half of Kenya's rare plants grow in the coastal region. Over fifty years of ever-growing demand for land and resources has dramatically reduced the size of *kaya* and has completely eradicated some smaller groves. Many factors play a role in the destruction, including population growth and expansion, the hotel and tourist industry, mining, agriculture, livestock, and the erosion of spiritual traditions. Knowledge of cultural values is declining, and thus they are pushed aside, often to the detriment of the holistic health of the community. The spread of Islam and Christianity had a negative impact as well.[6] Today, sacred groves and sites are gaining recognition once again for the vital role they play in biodiversity, sustainability, and conservation.

Early America's Tree Whisperers

Even in the United States, where enslaved Africans suffered what was arguably the greatest spiritual restriction and violent conversion to some form of Christianity, people found sanctuary for their spirituality amid the brush and arbors in makeshift sacred groves in America's deep forest. It was to the forest that early African Americans stole away to form congregations to sing and pray.[7] As the custom of tree talking demonstrates, we also maintained the custom of communication and learning based on tree knowledge.

OLD DIVINITY: THE STORY OF AN AFRICAN AMERICAN TREE WHISPERER

To learn *Jiridon*, the seeker, whether hunter, warrior, or shaman, must spend ample time alone in the wilderness, observing the workings of nature, including the expressions of animals and the whispered wisdom of the sacred wood. *Jiridon* studies are not carried out through an apprenticeship with a human; they are learned directly from trees and plants themselves. *Jiridon* meshes tree science with spirituality, and learning it can take a lifetime.

Ma gran'mammy brung tree-tawkin' from de jungle. Ah's from a tree-tawkin fambly, an' Ah ain't be livin' undah this watah oak evah since ah surrendah foh nuthin'. —Divinity

In early African American history there are accounts of people speaking the language of trees. Clearly those folk are masters of *Jiridon*. They were called tree whisperers. Tree whisperers in the United States spent time living with and studying a single tree. Living in total isolation from humans, within the forest or next to a lone tree, tree whisperers became highly observant. They listened attentively to the reactions of a tree to lashing wind and to sunny warm days. Eventually, tree whisperers heard trees speaking quite clearly to them. Trees teach those who will listen to be masters of *Jiridon*, master herbalists, and adept ecologists.

In 1930, Ruth Bass, a white Mississippian, collected a fascinating account of a tree talker in the Bayou Pierre Swamplands. It is an intriguing first-person account of this ancient practice. While Ruth Bass was very interested in early African American culture, some of her side comments reflect the cultural bias prevalent at that time, and yet her passion for the subject matter resulted in this very special story that will transport you to a different space and time:

> *In these swamp-lands I have often found traces of the old magic called tree-talking. Here magic becomes a still more imponderable thing and carries with it a philosophy that is more or less pantheistic. It had its roots in the friendship of the jungle man for the*

mysterious, animated, and beautiful world in which he lived. The swamp people, like the jungle men, recognize life in everything about them. They impart a consciousness and wisdom to the variable moods of material things, wind, water, trees.

Details are vague and hard to find, but, so far as I have been able to ascertain, the basis of tree-talking is the cultivation of a friendship with a certain tree—any tree of any species will do. It is simply magic, a magic that is still found in the Bayou Pierre swamp-land today. Among my acquaintances, I number one tree-talker. The other conjurers point to Divinity when I mention tree-talking. More than once I have visited his cabin on the edge of the swamp, burning with curiosity, and I learned nothing tangible. I resolved to try again and on a warm afternoon in autumn I followed the swamp path along the bayou until I found him—and what he lived by.

Old Divinity sat on the little front porch of his cabin at the very edge of the swamp. It was late October, dry and still with a low-hanging sky. Leaves were beginning to drift from the big water-oak that dominated his clean-swept yard. A frizzly cock and three varicolored hens scratched and clucked in the shriveled leaves under a fig tree near the porch. Six white pigeons sat in a row on the roof sunning their ruffled feathers. A brown leaf, whirled from the oak by a sudden gust of wind, fell on Divinity's knee. He laid a gnarled old hand on the leaf and held it there. A swarm of sulphur-yellow butterflies floated by. Silently, aimlessly, purposefully, they drifted eastward. Divinity sighed. *"Bes'tuh stay in one place an' take whut de good Lawd sends, lak a tree."* Here was my chance, it seemed.

"Yes, there's something of magic about a tree. I've heard that, for whoever can understand, there's a thing called tree-talking, ever hear of it, Divinity?"

"Did Ah! Ma gran'mammy brung tree-tawkin' from de jungle. Ah's from a tree-tawkin fambly, an' Ah ain't be livin' undah this watah oak evah since ah surrendah foh nuthin'." I felt that I was near to looking into that almost inscrutable Negro soul. Here were pages of precious folk-knowledge and all of it in danger of passing with ninety-six-year-old Divinity. What could I say to draw out a bit of his jungle lore? I said nothing.

The old man fumbled through his numerous pockets for his sack of home-mixed tobacco and clay pipe. A flame flared up from his match, and then the fragrance of burning deer-tongue slipped away in the soft air. Divinity rubbed his dry old hands together. I was afraid to seem too eager. Silence lay between us. Suddenly there came from the swamp pines and cypresses that crowded upon the little clearing, a soft murmur, a sound like the whimper of a company of comfortless creatures passing through the trees. We felt no wind and there was no perceptible movement in the treetops; but the gray swamp-moss swayed gently as though it was endowed with the power of voluntary motion.

"Heah dat? If yo heah murmurin' in de trees when de win' ain't blowin' dem's per-rits. Den effen yo know how tuh lissen yo kin git dey wisdom."

"Spirits of what, Divinity?" "Why, de sperrits ob trees! Dey rustle de leaves tuh tract tenshun, den dey speaks tuh yo." "So trees have spirits, have they?" "Cose dey does." The old man withered me with a glance, puffed out a cloud of fragrant smoke and proceeded, in his slow old voice, to tell me a few things about spirits. Everything has spirit, he told me. What is it in the jimson-weed that cures asthma if it isn't the spirit of the weed? What is that in the buckeye that can drive off rheumatism unless it's spirit? Yes, he assured me, everything has spirit. To prove it he could take me to a certain spring that was haunted by the ghost of a bucket. Now if that bucket didn't have a spirit where did its ghost come from? To Divinity man is only a rather insig-nificant partaker in the adventure called life. . . . To him it is stupid to think of all other things as being souless, insensitive, dead. "Is eberything cept'n man daid den? Dat red-burd yondah—" A cardinal, like a living flame, flashed into a dark pine. "Dat black bitch ob yourn—what she got?" Old Divinity hit home. I stroked the soft head the old spaniel rested on my knee.

Ruth Bass goes on to ask about the origin of Old Divinity's knowledge:

"It's a pity more men don't know this," I agreed, half to myself. "Yessum. It's a sho pity," Divinity agreed, half to himself. Then I asked Divinity how men could learn this truth of his. He assured me that some men were born with it, though most people had to find it out for themselves.

"What about you, Divinity, were you born with wisdom, or did you learn it?" "Me? Ah's de gran'son ob a witch," he answered proudly. "An' Ah's bawn wid a veil ovah ma face. A pusson what bawn wid a veil is er dubble-sighter." A double-sighter, he told me gravely, was a person who had two spirits, one that wanders and one that stays in the body. He was "strong in de haid." Divinity told me seriously, mixing great truths with sheerest fancy, he could see the wind. . . .

The sun was reddening in the west. A breeze had sprung up, bringing a continual soft murmur from the swamp trees. Old Divinity sat silent. His pipe had gone out. No wonder he sat and thought of death, so lonely and so old, with no one to look to.

"Do you get very lonely, Divinity, now that all your children are gone?" "No'm. When Jessmin, ma baby, lef', Ah felt sad at fust, but now Ah sets an' tawks tuh mase'f, er de trees an' de win'. . ." Bettah tuh stay in one place an' take what de good Lawd sen', lak a tree. . . . Dusk was creeping through the swamp. I rose to go. . . . Winter! Ah, win-ter, touch that little cabin lightly, I wished, as I turned through the darkening swamp, and left the old, old grandson of a witch sitting on his porch, while a lone killdeer

called up the wind. Mojo? Call it what you will. The magic of the swamp had come upon me. I found myself talking with the wind![8]

I never knew about tree talking or *Jiridon* as a child. Somewhere inside me, however, this Africanism lurked, and I heeded its call anyway.

ANGEL OAK

Old Divinity's affinity was with an oak and, as he says, there is "magic in the trees." In quite different American lowlands, there is a majestic oak called live oak (*Quercus virginiana*) that has become a part of the spiritual ethos of America's Gullah people. I had the good fortune to stay on one of the non-commercialized Gullah Islands called Edisto, where I drove down lush, tree-lined roads, and just so happened to get lost late at night in a forest where Spanish moss–draped live oaks dominate. The bearing of these trees felt ancient, primal, and terrifying at once. Often when we are lost, or when we've gone off the beaten track, we can truly surrender to the mystery and power of the forest.

Just a bit outside Charleston, there is a huge serpentine live oak on John's Island, South Carolina, called Angel Oak. Live oaks spread, rather than grow upward, so the tree is sixty-five feet tall and 160 feet wide, creating enough shade for 17,100 square feet. The tree branches go underground and resurface, lending it the distinctive air of a grove of trees, though in reality it is just one tree.

Angel Oak predates both the planter family for which it was named and the enslaved people whose spirits claim it as home. The tree is purportedly haunted by the souls of murdered African Americans who were lynched on the tree. Members of specific African tree societies were inevitably brought to the area and forced to work the land, cultivating "Carolina Gold" (rice). Some of them came to be known as Gullah people because of the unique customs and dialect they retained from West Africa. After lynchings, people who had the caul (a gift for seeing into the spirit realm) saw spirits around the tree. The deeply religious Gullah call these spirits angels. They pray and make spiritual offerings and petitions around Angel Oak; such is a common practice among some of our people in the Motherland as well as elsewhere in the diaspora.

Angel Oak can be visited free of charge. It is the oldest tree east of the Mississippi. Angel Oak is believed to be more than fourteen hundred years old.[9] If "Strange Fruit," the song hauntingly sung by Billie Holiday, makes your spirit ache, perhaps you should go pay homage to the spirits of enslaved and lynched black folk by making a discreet offering at Angel Oak.

Lessons of the Trees

Clearly, in both Africa and the New World, trees are commanding cultural reservoirs. The "first-born tree" is the seat of a community. The community grows and thrives along with that first-born tree. Its roots feed on spiritual strength and traditional values. Not only of spiritual value, sacred groves are a traditional African way of instilling and sustaining biodiversity. For example, baobab is a gathering place and shield, supplying food and water. Individual trees and groves are sacred because of their ability to shield a community from invaders while germinating medicinal seeds, pods, mosses, ferns, bark, and fungi. Sacred wood is home to insects, birds, reptiles, and other animals as well as to divine spirits and ancestors. Angel Oak, *Igboru-Egun*, *kaya*, and numerous other woods have ecological as well as social and religious functions in community health that cannot be underestimated. Encouraging, honoring, respecting, and protecting healing groves is both African custom and collective responsibility.

> *Encouraging, honoring, respecting, and protecting healing groves is a traditional African custom and a collective responsibility.*

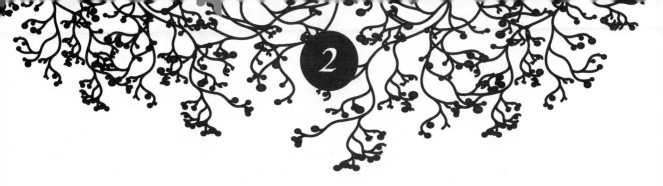

Calabash

VESSEL OF AFRICAN CULTURE, SPIRITUALITY, AND SURVIVAL

Calabash and the Lessons of Osayin

> *Top half of calabash is orun which represents invisible, spirit-realm where ancestors, goods and spirits dwell. Aye, its bottom half is tangible world. Creator Orisha, Odumare blessed both halves with ase (essential life force). Calabash represents the sum total of Yoruban cosmos.*[1]
> —Alisa LaGamma, Art and Oracle African Art and Rituals of Divination

Africans have a deep, abiding connection to trees of the sacred wood despite the brutalities and hegemonic thoughts about nature encountered during colonization. With the legacy of Osayin and his calabash, we now investigate tree lore, on both a cosmic and a microcosmic level, by visiting the spiritual world of *Ife*.

Ife

One of the most well known African Traditional Religions (ATRs) is the path of Yoruban followers of *Ifa*. This path touches me deeply because it preserves so much of African spirituality that sees the natural, human, and divine as being at a constant crossroad. *Ifa* stories are rich and varied. The corpus of this path helps us understand nature, human nature, and how the two relate. *Ifa* traditional medicine also enables people to become healers in a way that reflects African notions of health and how it intersects with community, ancestors, the creator, goddesses, and gods. Within *Ile-Ifa* is knowledge of all dis-ease, understanding of energy and its language, and access to natural, curative, protective, or preventive *ashe* (the magickal forces and energies of the universe) from wherever it exists, to bring about wellness.[2]

The Lessons of Osayin: From Africa to the New World

Devotees of *Ile-Ifa* throughout the diaspora believe that numerous orisha populate the world. Today the pagan community discusses about twelve orisha, but there are actually more than four hundred. Intimate contact with orisha brings dramatic change, difficult for science to explain. A curious orisha named Osayin happens also to be patron of the herbal arts. Unlike most other orisha, whose births are of orisha parents, Osayin sprang forth from the womb of Mother Earth herself as a sapling. Similar to a Tree Whisperer, living isolated within the wood taught Osayin all there is to know about plants.

*Ewe O, Ewe O
My plants, my plants!*

These days we would call this orisha "physically challenged." He is lame, with one arm, a very large ear that does not hear at all, and a tiny ear that hears extraordinarily well. This orisha has a screechy voice, difficult to listen to; thus he is associated with ventriloquism. Osayin is one-eyed and misshapen according to griots that teach oral traditions.[3]

He splendidly wears beads, which reflect the refreshing greens and blues of his forest. Birds and seeds, reinforced by the power of Ogun's metallic objects, play a role in his iconic representation, such as staffs. In Cuba and in American cities with a high African–Cuban American population, such as parts of Miami, New Jersey, and New York, Osayin's precious praise songs can be heard, and he is kept alive in botanicas through representative charms and forest medicines.[4] This complex orisha illustrates the end results of greed and selfishness and admonishes against hording natural gifts. His story is a cautionary tale to herbalists who become intoxicated with power, retaining it rather than sharing. It also reiterates the African tradition of healing medicine existing in trees.

We know Osayin as Green Leaf Man, Yoruban orisha of herbal medicines of sacred wood and bush, and patron of herbalists called *curandeiros* by African Brazilian people. Osayin is the orisha of wildcrafted herbs, berries, flowers, barks, and the entire wood. His presence has always captivated my imagination—he is the orisha at the center of my world.

Osayin collected all forest medicines and knowledge of how to use them. As a spiritual herbalist, he tucked all of his botanicals and knowledge into a *guiro* or calabash. There were numerous other helpful orisha, but Osayin wanted to keep knowledge of herbs out of their reach—high up in a tree, hidden.

Oya, orisha of weather and changes, generated a huge wind, followed by a storm that knocked the calabash of herbal knowledge down to earth. She did this with the blessings of orisha who desired herbal wisdom. This is a parable that we can use, and we have listened.

Osayin's devotees master taxonomic knowledge, studying leaves, herbs, and roots of the sacred wood. They learn to properly harvest, blend, and pound these tree medicines to create mind, body, and spiritual solutions. Incantations also known as *ashe* and *ase* are potent components of this healing methodology, because words yield power.[5] *Ashe* invokes spiritual power by tapping into the plant's liquids, whereas *ase* happens when a healer chews or ingests a power plant, then utters the incantations, bringing a double entendre to the magick. Incantations and the ability to divine bring this plant knowledge together, creating potent West African healing medicine.

The body of Yoruban myths of creation is called Odu. Odu includes the identification, uses, meaning, and secret words of plants. Moreover, every leaf on every type of tree has its own master. Herbalists who follow this path differ greatly from Western herbalists because spirituality is an explicit aspect of how plants can be used medicinally. There are rules for collection, uses, petitions, and offerings left for each tree of the sacred wood when Osayin sits on your head.

Osayin retains a very strong following in Cuba and Brazil, particularly western Cuba and northeastern Brazil. In Cuba, people who have retained strong ties to West African faith follow Osayin, and they connect him to the spirituality of the wood. The forest is called *el monte* (the mountain), because like a mountain it is filled with the awesome potential to heal. Osayin and creator are thanked for any medicines taken out of the wood, and offerings—typically herbs or blends derived from them— are left.[6]

Diviner's Gourds

Many different cultures in Africa use the gourd for spiritual or metaphysical purposes. For example, in the Democratic Republic of Congo, the Songye people of central and south-central Africa use *mboko* (gourd) in divination. Natural and man-made objects are put into *mboko*, shaken, and the configurations they take are interpreted. *Mboko* contains many different items that represent the natural world—for example, carved miniatures such as drums, collected organic matter such as bones, seeds, bird skulls, feathers, twisted vines, eggs, claws, animal teeth—especially of the lion and elephant—all inert until ignited by a specialist, called *nganga*.

The Luba people, also of central Africa, use gourd divination. *Kilemba* determines the guilt or innocence of a range of potential criminals.[7]

Gourd Healing in the Diaspora

In the Americas and Caribbean, there is an African-derived path (ADR) informed by *Ifa* practices called Regla de Ocha, or Rule of the Orisha. Osayin is represented by *guiro* (gourd) hanging in the *Santeria ile* (house temple). Tribute must be paid to Osayin before his herbal medicine can be used in ceremony or for spells, healing brews, potions, lotions, or balms. Osayin's symbols include the gourd where his spirit resides and the twisted tree branch where he hid healing knowledge and his colorful shades of green. In Catholicism, St. Benito, St. Jerome, and St. Joseph represent his spirit to those of the Christian faith.[8]

I am not on the path of *Ifa*; I am a practicing green witch (meaning I make magick and medicine with trees and other plants) and a hoodoo, focused on using that ADR path for its healing rather than harming potential. Still, as an African American I cannot help but look to this significant and distinctly African knowledge that *Ifa* represents to inform and enrich my healing work.

Healers celebrate natural cures, especially something as spiritually charged and full of possibilities as the calabash. We also realize that healing wisdom should not be constrained to a tight container and dispensed only by a powerful few. It should be available to all—this is the lesson of Osayin. Osayin's stash of herbal healing information, recipes, rituals, and ceremonies for health and spiritual well-being is as it should be—opened to all who come toward it in good faith.

Talk Fire Out of Burns: American Spiritual Medicine

The lessons of Osayin provide a lens through which we can understand the profound importance of herbalism and sacred wood to African healing, but this medicine manifests elsewhere in the diaspora. A tradition that seems to grow from *Ifa*'s *Odu* that could just as easily have stemmed from any number of Pan-African practices was recorded on the coastal plains of North Carolina, an area of our country that I might add has some unparalleled splendor created by the majestic, mist-kissed forests of the Blue Ridge Mountains. Mountains and foothills that start in Tennessee and bottom out in South Carolina will bring you to love and revere trees if you need some coaxing.

Mountains and foothills that start in Tennessee and bottom out in South Carolina will bring you to love and revere trees if you need some coaxing.

This area also hosts a unique form of faith healing; the power of words is used to heal. Ailments like burns are talked right out of the body! This practice, called Talk Fire Out of Burns, utilizes incantations for addressing angels. Just as incantations are commonly used in *ase* medicine, in *Ifa* and other ADRs, they are used by devout Christians in the southeastern United States for Talk Fire Out of Burns practice. These incantations invoke angels for healing. Here is one:

> *There came two angels from the north*
> *One brought fire; and one brought frost*
> *Go out fire and come in frost.*[9]

Talk Fire Out of Burns stems from direct communication with and understanding of the holistic nature of ailments utilized in West Africa by those who practice *Ifa*. Elsewhere in the diaspora, African-informed tree medicine is practiced by herbalists, medicine people, and a variety of healers. Their names in Jamaica are evocative, complex, and descriptive enough to let us know for certain: these specialists work holistically addressing mind, body, and spiritual realms. Apart from straightforward biomedical practitioners in Jamaica (of which there are plenty), there are also balm yard healers, mother healers, spiritual mothers, nanna herbalists, bush doctors, obeah practitioners sometimes called science men (who work magic sometimes using plants but are feared and not considered healers by many Jamaicans), psychic healers, revivalists, shepherds (and shepherdesses), brethren, and seers.[10]

Igbadu: Vessel of Divinity

Many important sacred and mundane tools are created from Osayin's calabash. *Igbadu* is a covered calabash that holds four smaller vessels, made from cocoa shells, cut in half, holding something unknown to the uninitiated. Two items derived from trees—charcoal and camwood—and two earth elements—mud and chalk—represent divinity. *Igbadu* loaded with these divine symbols are placed inside a wooden box called *apere*. The box is as sacred as its contents. It is used by those initiated into the ways of *Ifa*, and symbolizes divinity.

Vessel of Unique Sound

Art, dance, singing, poetry, and acting are not isolated activities in Africa or among other indigenous societies; they too can be brought into ritual, ceremony, or the individual healer's repertoire in an effort to forge change and bring wellness. The calabash has many uses in African holistic health, including art (especially music and dance) and divination; it is used as tool and implement as well as for stories that inform their creation.

In *The Healing Drum: African Wisdom Teachings*, authors Yaya Diallo and Mitchell Hall share soulful ways calabash are important to ceremony, ritual, and other community activities. Diallo reports that his people would not till, sow, weed, or harvest in fields without music. I know from doing Haitian and West African dance that every social and seasonal activity has a particular drum rhythm and dance. Dance and music accompany and enhance the work of farmers as well as fishermen, not to mention weddings, naming ceremonies, births, and funerals.[11] We know that the djembe (jembe drum) is made in large part from a hollowed-out tree trunk, but a few other stunning instruments are also created from calabash. These instruments have divine inspiration, a lengthy history, and an integral role in community health.

Balafon is an instrument of the spirit realm designed to communicate with the invisible world—*orun*, the inner dimensions of our universe. It is in the idiophone group of hand- and stick-played instruments, to which the xylophone also belongs, and it resembles one, however earthy, from the top. It has carved wooden keys mounted on a rectangular wooden frame. Strung underneath are a series of discreetly placed gourds with holes cut into their tops. The gourds act as resonators. Musicians hit the keys with two sticks wrapped with rubber ends. *Balafon* is a wind and percussion instrument. The tones have a quality that resonates with the water element in humans. Imagine the way rain and the sounds of a storm excite and soothe your soul; you are coming close to the intricate sound resonating from *balafon*.

Balafon's divine inspiration came from a dream. Sumanguru Kantey saw *balafon*, which did not exist in our world until he dreamed it. He heard its sweet music and awakened to create his vision. Kantey lived in the tenth century C.E., in what is now the Republic of Guinea.

Today, *balafon* is played during ceremonies—both religious and funerary—and is used to call snakes and reptiles. Because of its ability to draw snakes, *balafon* players wear protective amulets while playing in rural communities. To experience this music at home, try listening to the Balafon Orchestra, chaired by The Young People of Sara Kabba Tribe. They are featured in an eloquent CD called *Music of Chad*, which is commercially available.

Kora: Natural Voice of the Jeli

Kora is another instrument made from calabash, cut in half. It is a stringed instrument with a melodic tone resembling that of a harp. *Jeli*, called griots or storytellers by us, are revered musicians, usually brought into the art through musical family members, and in this way they are hereditary musicians. *Jelis* generally do not play *djembe*; instead, they play *kora*, *balafon*, *ngoni* (an ancestor of the banjo), and, today, guitar as well.[12] For *Jeli*, *kora* is the preferred instrument in Mali, whereas *balafon* dominates in the Gambia.[13]

Bafoko and Bolon: For Protection, Grief, and Ceremony

The music of Osayin's calabash is endless, and the Manding people put it to complex holistic use. They are attributed with independently developing agriculture between 3000 and 4000 B.C.E., and the country remains largely centered on farming.[14] *Bafoko* is a large calabash covered tightly with goatskin. In the middle is a circle of resin about four inches in diameter. The resin's location creates different tones. *Bafoko* is played in ceremonies along with *balofon*; the two were formerly played when warriors went to battle.[15]

A string instrument called *bolon* is based on *bafoko*. A stalk of millet is inserted into the skin of *bafoko* and is then attached inside a calabash. Two strings attach to the end of each millet stalk, rising above the skin and extending outside of the calabash. This has a bass sound when plucked. It is played at funerals and other ceremonies.

An ensemble cast, including Dembo Konte and Kausee Kuyateh, bring us the combined force of these instruments in *Jaliology*.[16] It's easy to see why these gourd-based instruments have been around nearly a thousand years, and why they are used in spirit possession festivals, ballets, and by the Komo Secret Society: they have harnessed that inexplicable energy that comes from the crossroads where nature, divinity, spirituality, and humans intersect.

Naturally, *jelis* would be able to pull off the feat of welding spiritual, divine, human, and natural, considering the divine origin of the instrument. Meanwhile, this telling of Osayin's story reminds us of hidden treasure—potentiality, in the ordinary looking, sometimes gnarly and ugly vessel he hid high up in the trees. His lesson asks us to look beyond appearances. Osayin's challenge is to see how many different helpful ways we can find for using one plant and its family. He asks us to look up to trees for surprises and even miracles. You'll find his symbolic calabash there, a truly remarkable vessel—swinging with the wind, pregnant with the possibility of numerous healing and household uses and making some of the sweetest music we can find on the earth, music designed with the specific purpose of touching the souls of humans, animals, and spirits. Through calabash we also understand our history in the Caribbean and the United States. It connects us back to Africa and our agrarian past.

Calabash: Container of Transatlantic Survivals

Not content to stay in Africa, calabash came right on over with us, figuring prominently in African American and African Caribbean history. That was plain enough to see when I visited Boone Plantation, outside Charleston, South Carolina. No, there weren't slaves; everyone there is paid now, but their spirit, paintings of them, photographs, and some of their possessions remain. It is one of few plantations with brick buildings, and, you guessed correctly, the enslaved created the bricks. But thanks to those brick slave quarters much was left intact, including simple handmade toys and even handprints. Seeing how little the enslaved families had, but how much they did with it, was very moving. There were handmade quilts and pottery, cast-iron Dutch ovens in fireplaces, and, not surprisingly, implements made from gourds. Still, their suffering was palpable, and if it were not for a Gullah man, hired as a griot, who creatively brought those tiny abodes to life using song, dance, and hand-hewn musical instruments, along with all the soul and spirit of his people, that visit would have been unbearable.

The calabash bottle gourd (*Lagenaria siceraria*) we saw reminds us how Africa was transported to the New World. It is symbolic of cultural survival. The bottle gourd is used as a float when fishing and this may explain how the gourd was able to establish itself across the Atlantic.

Jamaican enslaved people were given an extremely small allotment of personal goods during the early 1700s; one of these items was the calabash, which they used as a cup, bowl, spoon, and musical instrument resembling a lute. The other two items were a mat to lie on and an earthen pot for cooking. Calabash came to be used medicinally in Jamaica like a Chinese medicine method called cupping. The gourd was sliced in half, pressed hard on the painful spot, and removed briefly before the process was repeated.[17]

Thomas Jefferson reports in *Notes on Virginia* (1774) that enslaved people made banjos from large gourds with long straight necks on the plantations—they brought memories of *ngoni* with them. Another source reports that the long neck top was covered with rattlesnake skin, which would bring in some of the magical-spiritual *ashe* of the powerful snake.[18] This harkens back to instruments used to charm snakes (gourd instruments are used by Mande and other people of the area in snake ritual). This seemingly newfangled instrument was probably used in Virginia in ritual and ceremony as well. Creoles of color and black people in North America were reported to have used gourds as vases, goblets, and soup tureens. In fact, numerous groups of transplanted, enslaved Africans used gourds for water cups and bottles, and large gourds as storage jars.[19]

In Ghana and other parts of West Africa, the gourd is used to make spoons, ladles, and sieves, drinking utensils and a *danka*, which is a vessel for holding water, palm wine, and other fluids useful to the community. Following is a hands-on project for creating your own.

Calabash Vessel

The calabash is also used in ceremony, ritual, and ancestor veneration in some hunter-gatherer societies in East Africa. To create your own calabash tool try this project:

- ≫ Make a hole at one end.
- ≫ Pour boiling water inside to dissolve the pulp.
- ≫ Extract the pulp.
- ≫ Rinse with sand.
- ≫ Rinse again with water.
- ≫ Repeat until clean.
- ≫ Dry and then use.

Bottle gourds make great bird feeders and may also be used to make spirit dolls.

Pumpkins and squash were popularly used in the same manner.[20]

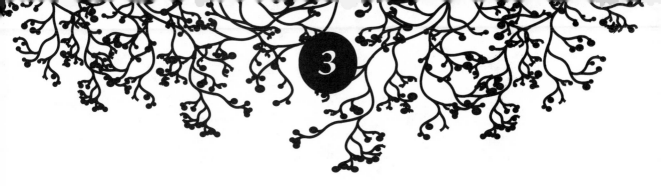

Black Folk Be Workin' Dem Roots Long, Long Time

AN AFRICAN HERBALIST'S OVERVIEW

> *Since the most ancient of times, African priests and priestesses and the common people believed in and used magic, medicine and religions to protect themselves from evil forces and to attract good ones.* —Camille Yarbrough, Female Style and Beauty in Ancient Africa

The Beginnings of African Herbalism

When I envision a distinctly African way of working with medicinal herbs, I look back to classical African civilizations. Within some of the earliest civilizations in Africa were vibrant cultures that revered all manner of healing trees and plants. This chapter examines herbalism and aromatherapy from ancient African civilizations to present-day African American and African Caribbean practices.

Today, herbalists use essential oils, hydrosols (flower and plant waters), and herbs for healing. All of these draw largely from medicines available in, on, and beneath trees. The use of aromatic trees, shrubs, herbs, oils, and waters therapeutically is called aromatherapy. This form of complementary alternative medicine (CAM) that integrates fragrance with health developed from Africa's ancient healing arts, and it is a sister to herbalism.

This story begins in ancient Egypt with Khemet, a high civilization of people still studied and admired. The Khemetian idea of healing establishes key features of holistic health and encapsulates what we know of African and diaspora healing elsewhere. I'm referring to a cohesive approach to healing, addressing the whole individual and his or her place within community. Facets of Khemetian medicine include examining environmental effects and combining arts such as dance, musical rhythms, correct attitude, and character with therapeutic plants, particularly from trees, and energetic stones. The potential cause of illness is examined holistically. Medicinal treatments include a variety of tree resins, gums, sap, bark, and leaves used as skillfully crafted incenses.

Fragrance of the Gods and Goddesses

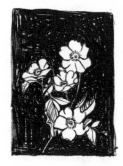

Early Egyptian priests practiced enfleurage, extracting aromatic oils from flowers. They also made numerous types of incense, some of which (for example, Kyphi) are still in use today. The early incenses were burned with spiritual intent, to please and come closer to gods and goddesses. Incense was burned at all important community ceremonies, including coronations of the pharaohs. Incense reigned in Khemetian temples, burning outdoors daily, marking dusk and dawn with blends of tree resins, saps, and herbs specific to gods and goddesses.

The Papyrus Ebers reports on the Khemetians' use of aromatic tree and herbal medicine, which combines fire and air as incense for metaphysical, magical, and healing purposes.[1] Hippocrates, known as the father of modern medicine, acquired most of his knowledge from the Egyptians.[2] Dioscorides, the Greek physician who created *De Materia Medica*, a document that set the standard for herbal knowledge, transcribed numerous African remedies and formulas.[3] Healing techniques utilizing fragrant plants practiced by Egyptians and other early African cultures fascinated the ancient Greco-Romans Pliny and Galen, who archived, experimented with, and passed down African herbal and aromatic healing formulas developed later in Europe.[4] In this way, African plant wisdom influenced Western herbalism and aromatherapy as they exist today.

One spectacular blend that has survived to the present day is Kyphi. Today, select alchemists still create these original Egyptian blends, but under the European names used by Dioscorides and Galen.

Africa's aromatic past is intriguing, and so is the continued engagement with and unique applications of aromatherapy in Africa and within the African diaspora. In some cases, herbalism simply means essential oils; in other cases herbs and aromatics in incense, rubs, pomades, solid perfumes, washes, baths, and floral waters are common applications used in Africa and the diaspora.

Lise Manniche states, in *Sacred Luxuries: Fragrance, Aromatherapy, and Cosmetics in Ancient Egypt*, that Egyptians noticed that the acacia possessed aromatherapeutic benefits because of its penetrating effect, even though its fragrance is subtle. Massage used acacia as an oil and poultice to help heal heart ailments. Manniche cites Coptic Africans as using this practice.[5] Copts are concentrated in Ethiopia, not Egypt, attesting to a collective knowledge.

Adama Doumbia and Naomi Doumbia, PhD, who write beautifully from a first-person perspective about Mande traditions, call acacia the *balanza* tree (*Acacia albida*), noting its potent stature in West African communities where the Mande live. The Doumbias say that *balanza* is a symbol of longevity and male procreativity and marks connection between the heavens and the earth. So auspicious is this tree that people don't rest under it without protection.[6] As you shall see shortly, there are many connections between traditions and reverence for plants between North Africa, our current focus, and West Africa.

Egypt, which many of us prefer to call Khemet, remains the most renowned ancient African culture. Khemetians used trees medicinally and spiritually for healing. They enjoyed exotic fragrant gardens, home to a variety of trees, and used fumigation and smudging for social events and in prayer, meditation, blessings, and healing—smudging was particularly noted for the treatment of women's reproductive ailments or discomfort. Even today, many botanical oils continue to come from what is now known as Egypt and other nearby countries.

Khemetians released plant essences into fixed oils through maceration, pulverization, soaking, burning, fermentation, water-based infusion, decoction, and the use of unguents. Khemetian applications still popular today include baths, rubs, massage, tinctures, poultices, body wraps, and teas, and what I would venture to call "hot toddies" (alcoholic herbal drinks).

The crossover between European and North African herbalism exists because many of the same plants grow in both regions and because renowned ancient physicians borrowed recipes and remedies freely. In *An Ancient Egyptian Herbal*, Manniche explains how Egypt could host herbs that we now enjoy in the United States, Europe, and the Caribbean.

Queen Hatshepsut and Exotic Botanical Gardens

Khemetians were fond of their gardens and went to great lengths to import plants from other parts of Africa, the Mediterranean, and the Middle East. One well-recorded venture was the effort by Queen Hatshepsut (1505–1485 B.C.E.) to transplant incense (frankincense and myrrh) from the Land of Punt to her temple in Deir el-Bahri, Egypt. There is a relief of Hatshepsut at Deir el-Bahri, from the eighteenth dynasty period, depicting the planting of numerous imported trees.[7] It is doubtful that the trees survived, as they still grow only in a very fixed geographic region that does not include Egypt; yet the effort demonstrates an early passion for gardening, and black women's early involvement with horticulture in Africa. Hatshepsut's successor Thutmose III tried to do the same thing, and his efforts are also preserved in art, capturing what is called "the Botanical Garden," probably the oldest recorded herbal garden.

Khemetians also designed an early permaculture system, enabling gardeners to irrigate newly planted trees and plants using the river Nile. Within their elaborate walled gardens, indigenous and imported fragrant, evergreen, and fruit-bearing trees and plants were interspersed.[8] Some examples of preserved art that can still be enjoyed in the present day showing the gardens include:

» Reliefs from the tomb of Meryre at el-Amarna, showing gardens at the Temple of Aten of the eighteenth dynasty

» A fresco of the Nursery Garden of Amun, in the tomb of Nakht at Thebes

» The Akhenaten and Nefertiti garden at el-Amarna (eighteenth dynasty)

Wholesome trees associated with North Africa such as pomegranates, dates, dom palm, moringa, argan palm, fig, and carob are intermingled with herbs such as myrtle and cornflowers, which we think of as being European, in the intact imagery of Khemetian gardens.

The sycamore tree, emblem of Hathor or Nut and Osiris, is also frequently shown in preserved art imagery. Even celery, an indispensable item in the American kitchen for stocks, stews, stuffing, and salads, is depicted in Egyptian art. Fragrant garlands created from celery leaves and blue lotus have been found on mummies dating from c. 1000 B.C.E.[9] Chamomile and lavender cultivars have also been found in pharaohs' tombs. Some of the earliest recorded history of perfume comes from Khemet. These cosmetics were made largely from aromatic trees. Khemetian perfume and beauty products feature tree resins, gum mastic, cedar, juniper, myrrh, frankincense, and pine.

First Still Developed by Maria Prophetissima

Like New York, Chicago, or L.A., back in the day Alexandria, Egypt, was *the* gathering place for experimentation, exploration, discovery, and creative thinking. A citizen of Alexandria during the first century C.E., Maria Prophetissima was an alchemist. Skilled in metallurgy, glassmaking, jewelry fabrication, pottery, and perfumery, Prophetissima created the first true still. It is nearly impossible to make good perfume or essential oils for perfume without a still. Called a *kerotakis*, her still helped the alchemist discover the essence of the body and spirit.

First Lady of Fragrance: Makeda, Queen of Sheba

You may have heard of Makeda, the queen of Sheba, through biblical references, the *Kebra Negast*, or the Koran. The romance between Makeda and Solomon, third king of Israel, is legendary. Their romance provides a snapshot of a delight in trees and herbal gardening and the role of both in the rituals and ceremonies of ancient African civilization.

Sheba was an empire centered in Ethiopia. *Ethiopia* in early Greek means "land of sunburnt faces." Ethiopian is sometimes a generic way of referring to brown and black people. In ancient times, Ethiopia referred to a wide geographical area, encompassing Upper Egypt and the African continent generally. Current-day southern Saudi Arabia, Yemen, southern Iran (Persia), and parts of India were considered Ethiopia.

Some scholars drew tighter boundaries, defining Ethiopia as falling below Aswan, Egypt, the Sudan, and present-day Ethiopia.[10] The queen of Sheba's empire included parts of Upper Egypt, all of Ethiopia, segments of Arabia, Syria, Armenia and India, and the region between the Mediterranean and the Erythraean Sea.[11]

The Kebra Negast (The Glory of Kings), a holy book written in the Ge'ez language, says that the queen of Sheba's empire was established in 1370 B.C.E. and lasted 350 years. This book also demonstrates a relationship between southern Arabia and Abyssinia (which is now called Ethiopia) in language, religion, and racial composition. This is supported by writings in Latin by Strabo and Pliny as well as a host of Egyptian hieroglyphics.[12]

The marriage between Solomon and Makeda was one of power. Makeda brought gifts to persuade King Solomon to enter into a trade agreement. Solomon became smitten with Makeda and had a crystal palace built for her visits; it was washed down completely in fragrant hydrosols, probably rose water, which was commonly traded in Persia and used for spiritual cleansing.

Carthage was another Ancient African empire involved with fragrant botanicals.[13] Carthage included present day Ghana, Mali, Songhay, and Kanem-Bornu.

The Land of Punt, also called Pwenet (*sacred land* or *incense land*), was prized for both incense and ebony. Punt was on the coast of Eritrea and Somalia.[14] Because of its geography and climate, Somalia remains a primary producer of quality frankincense and myrrh.

The gifts given to Makeda and Solomon for their wedding included sandalwood, cinnamon, cassia, attar of roses (rose water or oil), neroli (orange blossom oil or water), aloe vera, olive oil, sweet almond oil, and fragrant trees; in short, an array of healing gifts were brought, many of which came from trees and shrubs. The contributions to the nuptials demonstrate noteworthy international trade and cooperation and horticultural interests. Persian, Indian, Arabian, and West African botanicals were used by Shebaeans and are still used in contemporary Africa. This wedding highlights North Africa's spirit of cultural cooperation and its ability to learn from nearby cultures.

The marriage was one of many for the king—he is thought to have had over one hundred wives. In the end, Makeda left Israel, pregnant with their son, whom she raised alone. Imagining how the Shebaeans (offspring of Makeda) looked isn't difficult. Her son Menelik was the first king of the Solomonid line of Ethiopia, a line that ended with the deposition of descendant Haille Selasie in 1974.

The Yoruba Contribution

The Yoruban contribution to what we understand of West African herbalism is huge and cannot be overstated. These people from the great ancient Yorubaland Empire remain a vibrant culture. Often linked to *Ifa*, many of them are instead Christian or Muslim, the importance of which should not be overlooked to understand their full complexity. My friend Sharifa is a devout Muslim and would shun blanket identification with *Ifa* or other ADRs just because she is Yoruban. Another author friend, Nnedi, is Yoruba and Christian.

The Yoruba culture links our past to present-day herbal practices. Yoruban history begins with the migration of an East African population across the trans-African route, leading from the mid-Nile to the mid-Niger. Migrating Africans are thought to have used this route from remote times.[15] Michael Omoleya takes us back further: "The Nigerian region was inhabited more than forty thousand years ago, or as far back as 65,000 BC."[16] Olumede Luceus illustrates the point of connection between Egypt and sub-Saharan Nigeria: "The Yoruba lived in ancient Egypt during antiquity before migrating to the Atlantic coast." Luceus cites "similar languages, religions, beliefs, customs, and names of persons, places, and things." This is of interest to the discussion of African diasporic healing traditions because so many Africans enslaved in the New World came from Yorubaland.[17]

Meshing of North and West African Healing Vision

In volume 1 of his classic *Metu Neter*, Ra Un Nefer Amen states clear correlations between Yoruban followers of *Ifa* and Khemetic spirituality. For example, Ra Un Nefer connects the *Ifa* orisha and Khemetian deities with the same attributes, and lists the trees and herbs used to petition, call, and please them. Each Khemetian deity has spiritual baths, incenses, and herbal medicines that are used both to pay spiritual homage to the deity and for healing. In *Ifa*, each orisha has a corresponding herb, called *ewe*, and steep protocol as to how it is to be used. This way of fusing spirituality and health is not limited to the *Ifa* faith or Khemetian history; it is prevalent today in most ADR practice.

Jamaica's Holistic Healers

Nowhere in the diaspora is the amalgamation clearer than in Jamaica. To understand this, we need to peek into their ethnic history as it relates to Africa. Many Jamaicans attribute their African heritage to the Twi or Akan people. Some Jamaican words are closely aligned with Twi language, including *duppy*, which in Twi is *adope*, meaning spirit. There is also indigenous culture incorporated into Jamaica, courtesy of the Taino Native Caribbean people. Apart from Twi there is a recognized Kikongo contingent, also from West Africa. There is an East African connection to Haillie Sallasie. A helping of European blood from the British also exists, though there is also some contribution from the Portuguese and other cultures. There is a South Asian Hindu influence, and Jamaicans trace some of their heritage to China. Jamaican healers, and magic workers, whether they are considered obeah, myal, revivers, kumina, balm yard healers, or mother healers, consider the wisdom of ATRs, European herbalism, India's ayurveda, and concepts of Chinese medicine in their unique fusion of multicultural folk medicine.[18] This demonstrates why isolating Chinese medicine, ayurveda, and European herbalism as distinct makes no sense. African peoples have been living next to (and in some cases, with) and trading with these different groups of people for hundreds of years, particularly in places like South Africa and parts of the Caribbean. In the process, our healing practices are bound to rub off on one another, and it is from there that this knowledge is disseminated.

Quimbois: *Bain demarre and Bain de la Chance*

Many African cultures view the bathtub as a vessel for well-being. One such culture is *Quimbois*, practiced by Africans in French-speaking parts of the Caribbean. The two main types of therapeutic baths are *bain demarre* (bath to get rid of problems) and *bain de la chance* (bath to bring good luck). These types of baths are typically taken *plein air* (in the open air). A big earthen pan filled with water is placed under the sun. Magical herbs are added to the bath. With the heat of the warm Caribbean sun, a sun tea develops. Tree medicines and herbs used include paoca, calaba balsam, and bride's rose. Fragrant waters are ladled ritualistically over the head nine times by a healer, who also fills the water with the appropriate spiritual intent using prayer and incantation.[19] With its melding of herbal bath, numerology, and incantation, this Caribbean practice bears striking resemblance to American hoodoo.

American Rootworking

As a people, African Americans have traditionally communicated with and lived with other groups, and we continue to look at neighboring cultures for inspiration and for wellness information. Dr. Faith Mitchell's book *Hoodoo Medicine* highlights cooperation between African, Native American, and European cultures in the development of African American healing systems. Mitchell discusses the open-mindedness displayed by our people during challenging times, and our willingness to respect and incorporate traditions of others into our own corpus of healing. The blending of medical and spiritual dimensions in herbalism has been, and continues to be, an important hallmark of our culture.

My book *Sticks, Stones, Roots and Bones: Hoodoo, Mojo and Conjuring with Herbs* revolves around hoodoo, as it is the magical herbal tradition in the United States that embodies the essence of African healing wisdom with which I am most familiar. I will use the terminology of hoodoo, for example *rootwork* as a synonym for herbalism, because that is the way the practice has been described in the United States by African Americans historically.

Though initially it may elicit a flinch, the objective use of the phrase *witch doctor*, stripped of religiosity and negative stereotypes, aptly fits African herbalism as well, since it encourages spiritual and physical connection. A green witch knows her herbs, and she uses them to heal body, mind, and spirit in the same way that a doctor utilizes biomedicines to treat illness and dis-ease. The African American root worker does not simply heal a sore throat; she examines the environment, spiritual situation, and overall health and psychological state of her client before suggesting potential solutions.

I would like you to contemplate this quote by one of Africa's high profile and gifted community healers, who now lives in America. Malidoma Patrice Some is a Dagara originally from Burkino Faso; what he has to say crystallizes the motif of this chapter:

> For the Dagara people, the rain goddess, Sapla, is a tree. She is soaked with water, and should she dry up, there will be no rain for seven years. The roots of the tree and the plant are veins and arteries needing clean and nourishing water, which is sent upward to the rest of the body. This water must be pure, it must be real water, or it will not work. Our constitutions function in just the same way.[20]

Like a tree, we are one with nature and divinity, rooted with our ancestors, in a spiritually diverse global community. Without these aspects working in a clear partnership, nothing works and dis-ease shortly follows.

Past Is Present: The Art of Num

With the typical narrow historical scope of an American, until I researched my DNA ancestry I saw myself within the context of the last couple hundred years, centered in the New World, mired in slavery. The testing revealed that I am of the genetic haplogroup L1, and we are one of the oldest surviving haplogroups on the face of the earth. People in this group are mostly of African heritage, but the line extends into parts of the Mediterranean, such as Italy, Spain, and Portugal, as well as into Middle Eastern countries. The L1 lineage originates with hunter-gatherer peoples of South and East Africa, such as the Hadza, Khoi, San, and !Kung. I close this chapter investigating the original L1 ethos, visiting with !Kung to locate clues for the rich potential of combining seemingly divergent activities to yield powerful synergistic community health.

The Kalahari is a large basin of deep wind-etched sand in South West Africa. The basin covers an immense area, ranging from just north of the Gariep or Orange River in South Africa north almost to the equator. The southern Kalahari typifies the region, and it is often what is thought of as the Kalahari, though in reality the name encompasses a much larger area. The southern Kalahari is a dune-veld covering the crossroads of Namibia, South Africa, and Botswana.[22]

Kalahari peoples include the San, Khoi, Nama or Namaqua, Griqua, and !Kung people.[23] I want to focus here on the !Kung, a hunter-gatherer people who have always lived a difficult life, and things are only getting more politically and economically challenging for their people in the twenty-first century. Today they battle introduced diseases like HIV/AIDS as they fight to hold onto their lifestyle against all odds. As one of the few remaining hunter-gatherer groups, they experience prejudice and mistreatment from all Africans, regardless of color or ethnicity.

!Kung people live in different camps in the Dobe area of the northwestern Kalahari. Whereas we fuss and think the world will end if we have a "brownout" or—Goddess forbid!—a blackout, cutting our source of heat or, even worse, air-conditioning, !Kung live in harsh elements with barely an overhead shelter to keep out the monsoon rains or scorching sun. Traditionally, the only thing they cover is their genital area.[24]

One of the fascinating aspects of these people is that, despite their hardships, they have woven healing threads throughout the daily fabric of their lives. They make no division between sacred and mundane activities; their spiritual life is an inextricable part of their lifestyle. Every night is healing time, and this often involves trance and ecstatic dancing. !Kung do not have separate categories for sacred, ordinary, profane, art, herbal healing, shamanism, or spirituality; each of these facets come together cathartically, producing healthy results. Arts, divination, herbalism, and everyday life are entwined. In Western cultures, these are divergent practices suitable for neat categorization; in the Kalahari, all are tossed into the cauldron of !Kung, producing a rich stew that for millennia has sustained their culture. !Kung deities are as flawed as humans, and they contemplate their own betrayals, sexual antics, and needs up in the heavens.

GIRAFFE DANCE AS ALMIGHTY TREE

The tradition of healing in Giraffe Dance is like an almighty tree, sustained and nourished by the !Kung's hunting and gathering lifestyle, offering its fruits of protection and enhancements to individuals and the culture as a whole.[21]

!Kung people spend twelve to nineteen hours per week hunting and gathering food. There is much more gathering than hunting, and gathering is women's work. Sixty to 80 percent of their food consists of wild-gathered nuts, leaves, roots, fruits, and vegetables. They eat protein-rich and tasty mongono nuts, featured on page 99.[25] The mongono tree provides a major staple food in the !Kung diet. *Kameeldoringboom*, or camel-thorn-tree, grey-camel-thorn tree, Shepherd tree, *tsamma*, acacias, and yellow-flowered devils-thorn are also important to the Kalahari. At least two hundred other species occur there.[26]

They also dig various roots from the ground with handmade digging sticks, and, of course, they eat juicy Kalahari melon. By our standards, the !Kung of the Kalahari are deeply spiritual people. They call spiritual energy *num*. Not set aside for special occasions, or a specific day of the week, gathering and building *num* is a daily practice. *Num* is raised through dancing—dancing that sometimes becomes rapturous.

Ama Ama, healers of the !Kung, are revered. Prayers to deities can take place anytime, anywhere. !Kung speak plainly to goddesses and gods; their great god being *Goo Na* and the lesser one *Kautha*.[27] These deities live in the sky. Typical prayers are "give us your water (meaning rain)," "let food grow," and "give us a chance to rest."[28]

Sustainability Hinges on Community Cooperation

Desert heat and monsoonal rain demand sharing. There can be no hoarding of resources or food would quickly rot. Moreover, just as healing is an amalgamated practice, society itself is interdependent. If each group does not look out for all its members, they would be quickly wiped out by the elements.[29] !Kung gather at the water holes to catch up, telling the great stories and gaining much-needed sustenance. They relish the chance to share; they do it forthrightly and intentionally. Sharing is the cornerstone of their society—it is one of their most important seeds of hope passed down to us.

Looking across time and space from classical Khemet, Ethiopia, and Punt to modern-day Africa, which still sustains the !Kung and other original hunter-gatherer cultures, and newer blended African diasporic cultures of the Caribbean and Americas, our vision of health is without defined space or time. Mind, body, and spirit must be addressed to address the source of illness. Arts of music, song and dance, divination, shamanism, doctoring, tree medicine, and collaborative cooperation produce catharsis, which brings about synergistic healing. Wellness requires the acknowledgment of, and a spiritual unification with, nature. The root and gathering point was and still is beneath the trees.

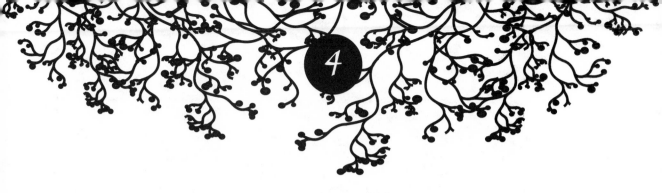

Ceremonies, Rites, and Oracles of the Wood

TRANSATLANTIC AFRICAN TREE VENERATION

I'm not quite sure where or how, but we brought our belief systems with us, though our cord seems to have been brutally severed from the Motherland. Nothing makes this clearer than looking at our transatlantic relationship to trees. We observed the healing ways of indigenous people in areas where we were transplanted, but the development of African diasporic ethnomedicine was not taught to us; rather, what we knew went through some form of adaptation, also noted in other immigrant groups. By and large, we developed our healing ways in the New World through experimentation, testing, and direct observation, as has been the way of herbalists and shamans around the world from time immemorial.

The notion of sacred trees offers a good example. *Iroko* (*Chlorophora excelsa*) is one of the most respected spiritual trees of Brazil, inspired by *Oloko*, the sacred silk cotton tree of West Africa. In Candomblé, *Oloko* represents the god of time and eternity, since he resides within the tree. The male deity of time is also associated with peace, settling disputes between humans. Temples were built wherever this tree grew. New World *iroko* germinates spontaneously, growing quick and strong where other trees take their time, lending it more mystique.

This approach to trees harkens back to Yoruban liturgical plant taxonomy; conceptually, though sharing some resemblance to Native American ways, it remains distinctly African. The

---

KOLA NUT

The kola tree is *C. nitida*, yielding kola nuts. A sweet beverage called *bese* is made from bitter cola. Kola is indigenous to the forests in Ghana and cultivated in Sierra Leone and the Niger estuary in Nigeria. The nuts of *C. nitida* are the richest source of caffeine, and its stimulant ability is one of the nut's major uses. Kola has been exported from Ghana since prehistoric times to the northern savanna regions. Kola was once an ingredient in Coca-Cola, although the flavor and stimulant each come from different sources.

Kola nuts are sacred to Obatala, the old wise one, and Shango, the thunder orisha. Palm is used as an offering to the trickster orisha Elegba, while the warrior orisha Ogun desires palm wine and oil. Nut divination typically supplies yes or no answers, though more complex readings are sometimes given.

Yoruba evaluate medicine primarily based on the sensory attributes of the tree: what it does, how it appears, how it grows and moves, and its countenance, smell, and feel.

Professor Robert Voeks provides an intricate analysis of the Yoruban relationship to the forest and its development in New World Brazil in *Sacred Leaves of Candomblé*. According to Voeks's work, the belief system the Yoruba brought with them to Brazil was African to the core. Reverence and meaning are attached to sacred places and parts of the land, including villages, hillsides, mountains, rivers, ocean, stones, and—our focus here—the forest and specific trees.

Voeks calls the Yoruban belief system myopic and describes it as a closed and fixed religion, where close inspection to the details of the land dominates. Enslaved Africans in Brazil successfully introduced one of their sacred trees, the *obi* (*Cola acuminate*), for example.[1]

While there is a similarity between climate and terrain in Brazil and West Africa, not all spiritually significant plants could be transplanted. Substitutes were made and new plants added to the corpus of African Brazilian medicine. For example, the Brazilian substitute for African *iroko* is usually *Ficus spp* or *Gameleira branca*. Both trees are in the mulberry family, and both bleed latex when cut. They are formidable, broad, commanding trees, with multiple niches and buttresses, just right for placing offerings to spirits, ancestors, and various deities. Latex from the *iroko* has many medicinal applications, including the reduction of swelling and tumors.[2]

Ficus: Tree of Freedom

When I took you into my personal forest at the beginning of this journey, I related the way the ficus had served as my tree of hope when I lived in a Latino community that was deprived of any substantial presence of trees. My tree was a relatively small, potted indoor tree. Any trees can be important, whether you are living in a loft, apartment, or other nonrural dwelling. Ficus, my tree of choice, also known as fig, grows easily in most interior spaces. I have seen some reach fifteen feet or taller in indoor mall atriums.

FREDERIKSTED BANYAN

Frederiksted Banyan was an enormous ficus near the Fisherman's Market of Frederiksted, St. Croix, and it too held the hopes of a people. Like many sacred trees of Africa and the New World, ficus, or banyan as it is sometimes called, has numerous tangled roots and a tall dense crown and is a favorite gathering spot for both humans and spirits such as *Jumbie*. During enslavement, medicine men and women, also called "weed people" by islanders, gathered around this particular ficus, chanting and dancing before its

> Trees in the form of houseplants help fight indoor air pollution. A preliminary study by former NASA scientist Dr. Bill Woverton suggests that trees as indoor plants absorb contaminants in the air. Plants are considered helpful in removing formaldehyde, benzene, and carbon monoxide from indoor living space.[3]

massive roots system in "Jumbie congregations" designed to invoke spirits, petitioning for their help with gaining freedom from enslavement. Sadly, this celebrated island tree was destroyed during Hurricane Hugo in 1989.[4]

Libaka of the Ngome: Tree of Covenants

To understand the process of transatlantic folklore transmission and nature spirituality in the African diaspora, one of the most fascinating trees to explore is the silk cotton tree. *Libaka* is the name for the silk cotton trees used by Ngome people of the Democratic Republic of Congo (DRC). *Libaka* is a sacred tree that symbolizes the union of seen and unseen worlds. It is where a living community converges with ancestors.

While a new village is being established, it cannot become an official living space until the chief plants *libaka*. At the end of the first hunt, each hunter cuts a special stick that he plants in the ground, close to *libaka*. The sticks are all tied together with a special cane, which is fixed with seven knots. Knotting is a cross-cultural technique that serves a powerful and symbolic ritualistic purpose. Numerology is also important to us in Africa and the diaspora. We use the two specialties in various healing and magickal practices.

Libaka is treated with respect. Two important covenants associated with this tree are peace and friendship. It is essential that these agreements be made at *libaka*, for then the ancestors witness, participate, and share in the covenants.[5] Elsewhere in West Africa, silk cotton trees are dressed with a ring of palm leaves around the trunk, an offering to various orisha.

SILK COTTON TREE

Libaka is the silk cotton tree (*Ceiba pentandra* [L.] *Gaertn*) , a native of South America that has spread to primary rainforests of West Africa and parts of Asia. It goes by many names, including the *Ceiba* (pronounced "say-ba") tree. This tree holds a lofty position in West African and New World healing medicines. It is a massive, rapidly growing deciduous tree, capable of reaching over eighty feet—in some regions up to two hundred feet—in height. Its diameter is a massive five to eight feet above its buttresses. No small fry, the buttresses extend up to ten feet tall and can continue ten feet from the trunk. Large spines grow from the trunk, discouraging damage and inviting spiritual awe.

This community tree houses many aerial plants, insects, birds, frogs, and other animals and plants that use its height to obtain sunlight. The silk cotton tree produces three- to six-inch long elliptical fruits, which contain numerous seeds encased in a dense mat of cottonlike fiber. The fibers are dispersed like downy snowflakes into the air when the fruit ripens. The fibers are largely made of cellulose; light and airy, they are resistant to water penetration, with a low thermal conductivity. Silk cotton tree fibers cannot be woven, so they are used as a stuffing fiber, to insulate, pad, and create life preservers, as well as for stuffing mattresses and pillows. The oil is very useful for cosmetics, massage therapy, and hair and skincare.

KAPOK: NATIONAL TREE OF PUERTO RICO

The silk cottonwood tree is called *kapok* in Puerto Rico, where it is the national tree. The tree has been planted in many plazas for shade, and it is valued as a honey tree. Puerto Rican practitioners of Santeria, a faith inspired by Yoruban beliefs, use the tree in their rituals in six ways:

>> Leaves are used in love magick.

>> Offerings and sacrifices are placed at the roots.

>> The trunk is used for hexing and curses.

>> The bark is used medicinally in brews and potions.

>> The soil where the tree grows is used in magick.

>> Its shade attracts the spirits, lending supernatural power to those buried beneath.

JAMAICAN TREE OF THE DUPPY

In Jamaica, many different types of spiritual practitioners believe that spirits of the dead, called *duppies*, live mostly in silk cotton trees. The tree is not to be planted too close to home, because the *duppies* who live in them have an otherworldly temperature, and their heat brings discord to people. *Duppies* can be good or bad, but the most noticeable ones are temperamental and mischievous, and can hurt people if disturbed. *Duppies* live in and around silk cotton trees, which are called Duppy Trees, and in Duppy Coconuts and Duppy Cherries. Like the free-form silky tufts of cotton carrying seed, *duppies* drift off the silk cotton tree, making their way into nearby cities, towns, and farms. One can feel the *duppy* presence as heat passing through the body; once the heat rises, it's time for a healer to provide cooling medicine to bring the all-important balance back to the *duppy*-struck individual.

JUMBIE SPIRIT TREE OF THE VIRGIN ISLANDS

Similar to *duppy* spirits, but with their own unique quirks, *jumbies* are spirits that live at the roots of the silk cottonwood tree, called *kapok* in the Virgin Islands. Kapok is seen as a primarily spiritual tree—a holding place for the departed. Eggs are thrown at kapok when necessary, to free a person's shadow or soul stolen by *jumbie* spirits from being held by the tree.

CEIBA OF CUBA

Cuba, a part of the West Indies, is situated in the Antilles Archipelago. Many Africans were enslaved and brought to Cuba, to work the fields as slaves. Cuba has nearly three thousand endemic plants. The silk cottonwood is called *ceiba* in Cuba, where it grows well. *Ceiba* has an important role in Cuban spirituality. African Cuban followers of the *Ife*-inspired Lucumi form agreements, make petitions, and do invocations, rituals, and ceremonies beneath *ceiba*.

KAPOK AND THE MAROONS OF SURINAME

In Suriname, there are people called Maroons who had quickly escaped their captors before they could be enslaved.* These people retained a great deal of the social traditions, communal customs, and healing ways of sub-Saharan Africa. The traditional medicine of Surinamese people includes many uses for the silk cottonwood tree, which they also call *kapok*. *Kapok*'s seeds, leaves, bark, and resin are used to treat asthma, dysentery, fever and kidney disease. Its tree medicines are also used for the regulation of menstruation.

WEST AFRICAN SILK COTTONWOOD MEDICINES

Called *onyina* in Ghana, silk cottonwood bark has several medicinal applications there.

» A bark decoction is used as an emetic.

» A bark infusion is used as a fever remedy.

» Combined with jatropha oil, it is used to create healing ointment for sores and wounds.

» A decoction of *onyina* root is used to treat leprosy.[6]

Tamarind

Another sacred tree in Africa and the diaspora is the tamarind. This tree's metaphysical ability was well established in the nature veneration of Carib Indians, the original people of the Caribbean. Then, from the seventeenth through the nineteenth century, enslaved West Africans were brought to the West Indies, bringing their own tree-related beliefs.

The tamarind is revered. It has a supernatural bearing and feathery foliage, suggestive of the spirit world. The tamarind was introduced to the Virgin Islands during the colonial era when enslavement was also prevalent. The fat trees produce very deep shade. In Ghana, tamarind bark is chewed to relieve hiccups.

The tamarind is called *taman* tree. A celebrated tamarind called Tallo exists on St. Thomas Island. On the islands, *taman* is known as a gathering space for good and bad spirits. Children are told: *Don't sit under a tree after six P.M. or lean up on the tree, especially near a graveyard, or a* Jumbie *will follow you home. You will feel the heat. You get hot, that's how you know a spirit is in the vicinity.*

---

*Maroons have a sizeable presence in Jamaica as well.

≫ The dead have been interred in its hollowed trunks, which can create the right environmental conditions for natural mummification.

≫ It shares an elevated position in folklore and holistic health with the silk cottonwood, and is a relative of that sacred tree.

≫ It is one of the primary sustenance trees of hunter-gatherer peoples of South and Southeast Africa.

Rites of Passage

The baobab has been utilized in birthing ritual and death rites. The tamarind helped transport people metaphysically back to the Motherland. Middle passage, birth, and death are all types of difficulties these trees have eased. African trees also play a role in other rites of passage.

Women experience their blood vividly from the onset of menarche until menopause. Each month, we see evidence of the power and mystery of creation flowing from between our legs. To Yoruban medicine people, this is the hidden secret of red manifest. Menstrual blood is examined for its health and used in ritual. It is not considered a dead or useless substance, as it tends to be from a Western biomedical view. In Yoruban medicine, ideal menstruation is a health indicator. Its color, duration, texture, and scent is examined by healers and called *pupa daadaa*.[16] Not surprisingly, we have a cache of herbs to address various elements of our blood passage in African traditional medicine and those practices inspired by it.

The Beauty Way in Matters of Initiation, Life, and Death: The Sherbro Yassi Secret Society

Sherbro ideal beauty exudes cultivated refinement; health in mature womanhood is depicted in sculptural objects as having elaborately designed coiffure, bright, shiny, luminous black skin, and a long neck accentuated by neck rings.

CAMWOOD

Camwood (*Baphia nitida*), a deep red wood, plays a significant role in West African health and rites of passage. Because red signifies good health and vibrancy, red wood

A three-hundred-year-old tamarind near the National Guard Armory on St. Croix is called Emperor by local Rastafarians. Emperor presides over more than two dozen graves. Earlier on I mentioned how early African American graves typically include trees to connect the living with ancestors, and nature as well. In fact, in both Africa and the diaspora, specific trees such as the tamarind are designated community gathering places; and they became meeting places for the enslaved who sought emancipation. Later, union workers met to hash over labor issues there. Sacred trees such as the tamarind also serve as ancestral shrines; portals to our ancient homeland are found within special types of trees. Slaves entered trees' hollows to escape the harsh realities of the New World, choosing instead to be transported back to the Motherland.

Trees like the tamarind can be repositories of healing or curses; *Jumbie* spirits live at the roots of certain trees, including the tamarind.[7]

HABIT, GROWTH, AND DISTRIBUTION

As a botanical specimen, the tamarind is a beautiful yet ornery tree. It can grow as easily in semiarid as monsoonal climates. It is a productive fruit-bearing tree, and it manages to thrive through the six- to eight-month drought periods that are common where it has established itself. The tamarind actually produces more fruit when there is less rainfall. It is, however, not tolerant of lengthy cold temperatures, or even a brief frost. The tamarind originated in East Africa's Madagascar. Arabs spread the seeds, establishing it elsewhere.

TAMARIND'S FRUIT: GOOD EATING

Tamarind fruit makes bittersweet sauces for curries, syrups, and processed foods. Tamarind pulp is added to curry dishes, chutney, preserves, pickles, sherbets, and beverages. My favorite Middle Eastern sauce, lal chutney, is created from tamarind. Most people come across tamarind frequently, whether they realize it or not, as tamarind is an important ingredient in A1 steak sauce and Worcestershire sauce.

Though it may be hard to find in a regular grocery store, today you can find tamarind in health food stores, grocers who specialize in organic foods, and in Mexican or Latino *supermercados* or *fruterias*. I bought a pack this morning for less than a dollar. I have grown partial to it. It looks like pods with a soft, suedelike, medium-brown skin. If you peel open or crack the skin (sometimes it is brittle), there are flesh-covered seed kernels inside. Peel off the outer fibers (there will only be one or two and they are hard to miss), and then just suck the fruit from the kernel. They are pleasantly bitter and sweet and reminiscent of the old-fashioned candy Now or Later, without the empty-calorie guilt or worry for your teeth.

INTERNATIONAL USES FOR TAMARIND

The U.S. pharmaceutical industry processes one hundred tons of tamarind pulp annually. Tamarind fruits are used to reduce fever and cure intestinal ailments. It is well documented as an aid against scurvy because of the vitamin C it contains. It is a common ingredient in cardiac and blood sugar–reducing medicines.[8] The pulp is being used more frequently in commercial botanical-based skincare. The wood is hard and dense and burns well as charcoal. Tamarind wood also comes to a brilliant polish and is used in furniture making.[9]

The tree is adaptable, productive, communal, mystical, and supernatural. The metaphor set up by its fruit, which produces bittersweet sauces, confections, and dishes, is especially poignant. Bittersweet tamarind is a reminder of life during enslavement and the time shortly after emancipation in the Caribbean and the Americas. The tamarind has moved deftly across borders, serving our transatlantic culture well, and should be respected as one of our chief holistic healing trees.

Baobab: Anchor of the Savanna

The baobab has such a rich reservoir of mythology, folklore, and communal medicine that it has become emblematic of the Motherland. One story of the Khoi and San people states that when each animal was given a special tree during creation time, the hyena was bestowed with the baobab. Disgusted by the odd appearance of the baobab, an angry hyena threw the baobab tree down to earth and it landed upside-down. This offers an explanation for its strange appearance. Baobabs are frequently called the upside-down tree because their branches are spindly and gnarled and look like roots rather than branches. The tree is also called the lemonade tree because of an acidic beverage made from it, and cream-of-tartar tree or tartar tree because it contains tartaric acid.

> *When the universe was made, baobab was the last tree created.*[10]
> —*Island grandmothers, Virgin Islands*

BAOBAB AT ESTATE GROVE PLACE, ST. CROIX

While we in America tend to think of the baobab as situated firmly in the Motherland, that is not entirely the truth. In the Virgin Islands, at Estate Grove Place, St. Croix, grows the largest tree of the West Indies, a baobab that is fifty-three feet high

and fifty-three feet in circumference, with a sixty-seven-foot crown spre lore states that people have hidden in the huge hole in the trunk during h women have given birth there. It was the helm of uprisings and locus of me transports to Africa.

These fascinating trees (*Adansonia digitata*) are one of the only species on the savanna in Africa, accentuating their reputation for being bizarr seem out of place even on their home turf. Baobabs grow in arid, semiarid humid tropical climates.[11] Extremely long-lived, a baobab's lifespan is be thousand and three thousand years. *Jumbies*—spirits of the undead—love the baobab.

HEALING FROM THE BAOBAB

In addition to being a metaphysical and socially significant tree to the c the baobab holds very important biomedicines. The seeds of the baobab pulp with numerous uses. The vitamin C content of the fruit averages grams per 100 grams, nearly six times higher than an orange.[12] The bao also rich in vitamins B1 and B2 and phosphorous, iron, trace minerals, a Because of their iron and vitamins, the leaves are used in Ghana's traditi cine to treat anemia.[13] It contains essential fatty acids (EFAs) and polysat acids (PFAs), lending medicinal and food value. Baobab oil is useful f and cosmetics. The nutritious oil has a faint aroma, making it suitable f oil and other natural products. Baobab has a long shelf life, making it international shipping and storage.[14] I have found it to be a comforting, u skin treatments to deter the appearance of wrinkles, and to condition my soften rough skin at heels and elbows, and soothe dishpan hands.

Baobab's Key Features

≫ It is used as a gathering place in the community, even functioning as café and meeting room inside the hollow trunk.

≫ It can be used as a water reservoir.

≫ It is resistant to drought.

≫ Its seeds provide valuable oil.

≫ The pulp is rich in vitamin C and other nutrients.

≫ Island women have given birth in holes in the trunk; local traditions that people have ridden out hurricanes there as well.[15]

is rubbed on the skin to exfoliate and beautify, bringing out highly valued ruddy tones, signifiers of African women's health. One piece of Yassi Society sculpture is the *Female Figure with Tray Base*, done in current-day Sherba Island, Sierra Leone. The land of Sherbro, Kanwo, and Sitwa chiefdoms illustrates this desired quality of the skin in high art. This particular piece was collected between 1936 and 1937 by the University of Pennsylvania Museum of Archaeology and Anthropology, Philadelphia, where it remains.[17]

In this type of women's secret society, "medicine" means power and the knowledge to decipher, diagnose, and bring about changes, powers owned by diviners called *theng no* by the Sherbro people. Sometimes this means *theng no* have the task of figuring out what is just punishment for criminal acts called "witchcraft" in this part of Africa. *Thengo no* hold Sherbro's *materia medica* concerning the natural and supernatural world and its role in the community. These women know all the antidotes to poisons affecting mind, body, or spirit.

The Sherbro Yassi society figure I speak of was a noted guardian—a glowing, idealized black woman placed in a bowl, in front of a "medicine house." Supreme figures in this society are called *behku mama*; below them in rank, but still VIPs, are *yamama*. These healers' workings are similar to Mende practices, wherein mental health and agrarian fertility are seen to by female diviners who belong to secret societies.[18]

Sherbro figures are used when new initiates to the society are brought before the community, or when a society member dies.[19] This idealized beauty, with luminous skin, elongated neck, and fierce cornrows represents spirit mediating on behalf of the "medicine." They also show the community key symbols of health through trees like camwood. The figure is anointed with oils, furthering its desirable appearance in its lustrous, shiny skin. Whereas shiny hair is one of the most celebrated features of just about every other culture, vibrant, glowing, or red-toned skin, a distinctly African quality noted in our figurative sculptures, survives and thrives among Africans. To this day, "ashy" (dried or white in appearance) skin is frowned upon by African-descended people across the diaspora.

RED SKIN MEDICINE #1

Red palm oil is used in African massage to improve circulation and raise color. Red palm oil, like camwood, has an immense spiritual dimension.

Red tone can be evident in all healthy African-descended complexions, from the fairest to the darkest hue, and is not limited to one or the other.

Throughout the diaspora, types of tree medicine that are used on skin and hair to achieve desired effects include cocoa butter, coconut, banana, shea butter, babassu nut oil, and mango butter, to name a few. For adding a metaphysical dimension, red camwood is still ideal. Camwood has strong colorant strength, symbolic of safety and concealment, two significant features of Yoruban medicine—features carried over to New World secret doctoring.[20] Without a doubt, we like red.

Red During Nuptial Rites

In parts of sub-Saharan Africa, impending weddings are a time to celebrate a fresh, new, provocative stage in a woman's life. During her prenuptial period, the bride-to-be is elevated to a position of royalty. While our bridal showers are a one-day event, young West African "queens" are lavished with gifts and treated to indulgent natural beautification recipes over an extended period.

In many parts of Africa, betrothal is reminiscent of the limbo between life and death. There is dread of what the young woman may suffer, fueled by unpredictable outcomes. The bride-to-be is encouraged to gain weight so she appears sturdy and capable of bearing many children, quite unlike the American tendency to diet and shed pounds before weddings. While most folks shy away from intentionally packing on additional pounds, the idea of taking time out to be spoiled should be required medicine.

For African-Caribbean brides trying to incorporate "roots culture" in their nuptials, a skin and body type idealized from ancient Nubia, Punt, and Khemet to present-day South and West Africa is worth consideration. Put the face powder down; it makes us look ghostly. Listen to the numerous blues and hip-hop songs celebrating "thick," "apple-bottomed," or "big-boned" women—walk on, stand tall, and be proud.

In West Africa, the entire village gathers to sing praises and blessings for the marriage that is about to take place. The bride-to-be is taken to a small hut, and she stays there until her husband joins her. Her husband bestows gifts upon the community, and usually the marriage is consummated. The

RED SKIN MEDICINE #2

When ground and made into a paste, camwood is left on black skin or on braided or tightly curled or cropped hair—spiritual makeup, if you will—leaving the wearer with a red-coated, otherworldly, and potent yet provocative appearance. You've probably seen photographs in *National Geographic* or *Women of the Ark Calendar* of camwood applied to men or women, perhaps not knowing that it was tree medicine with which they were painted.

next morning a goat is sacrificed; its red blood is poured as a libation on the threshold of the hut. If the bride reports to her mother that she is pleased by her husband, dancing and celebration ensue.

People offer money for the pleasure of either visiting with the bride or rubbing her body with camwood, enhancing her desirable red skin with its natural dye. Camwood is a traditional symbol of good fortune because of its red tree medicine. Camwood rubbed on the skin encourages rejuvenation by removing dead skin, replacing it with a wholesome glow. Considered restorative, camwood brings a healthy complexion to all ages. Reddened skin balances the blood, so that there is not too much bitterness held within.[21] Whereas we throw white rice, red blood is the preferred offering in many parts of Africa. Goat blood libations, in particular, offer couples similar gifts to white rice—blessings, good fortune, and fertility.[22] All this centers around the nature of red, implicit in a tree like camwood.

Red Tree Oracle

Deeper into the forest is a fascinating culture: the Apagibeti are hunters and horticulturalists living in the rainforests of north-central Zaire. They tend plantain, manioc, corn, and peanut crops and hunt or trap antelope, monkey, pig, buffalo, and elephant. Village life is active. During June rains, men move out to the bush to set their traps and hunt. They remain in the wilderness seven months, returning only to carry dried meat to feed their community. For the Apagibeti, the main problem in life comes when the forest closes up.

They have developed a unique form of divination called *lekeye paye, wukeye paye* ("wakening the forest" or "opening the forest"), using leaves from a red-barked tree to figure out how or because of whom the forest came to close up, and to figure out how to reopen it. As occurs in several ATRs and ADRs, the creator *Nyombo* or *Njambe* is well respected but rather remote. It is ancestors who intercede in mundane and spiritual life, ensuring fertility, reliable food crops, good hunting, and successful social relations. At the ancestral shrine, offerings of kola nuts are left to ancestors.[23]

Three types of people adversely affect the hunt, thereby affecting village society generally: twins, witches, and *mangodo* (people whose top teeth erupted before the bottom). *Yingo*, forest spirits, are not feared; after all, the Apagibeti live in accord with the forest, so forest spirits are not something to fight, but something to embrace. They fear sorcerers most of all.

Apagibeti believe *paye awukisi basu*, "the forest saves us."[24] However, the wood can only serve as food source, refuge, and abode if it is kept open. One way to keep the forest open is a fascinating form of tree-based divination. Here we see an entirely different type of boiling energy, in a different ecosystem within Africa, used for the greater good of the community.

In *Mbolongo* divination, a man, not necessarily a shaman or divination special-ist, cuts red wood scrapings from the *mbolongo* tree's bark. At dawn the next day, he combines the scrapings with water in an earthenware pot over a fire. (Someone might dance the spirit of animal[s] they wish to kill.) The diviner covers the top of the earth pot with *ngongo* leaf and seals it with string wrapping that goes from the top to the bottom of the pot. He then draws three trails out from the fire, which appear as spokes of a wheel, while addressing the oracle with a question. The ques-tion is about who or what closed the forest. The focus is on whether an unknown pregnancy, an unknown or impending death, or the unknown eating of a first kill by *mangodo* (witchcraft or sorcerer, synonymous with evildoers in this society) closed the forest.

When the pot has boiled long enough, its leaf cover splits, and boiling *mbolongo* mixture teems down to the earth, radiating out along the spoke lines; this trail reveals the cause of the misfortune.

Some mixture is carried in a leaf shaped like a cone by a diviner or a child to a hunting net site, and the remaining brew is taken to where the diviner squats, wait-ing in the forest. With his back to the forest, he hurls the potion over his shoulder toward the village, stands up, and walks back into the forest.

Forest people probably live closest of all humans to the energy of the sacred wood. They know and value its goodness, as reflected in their proverbs, actions, and divina-tion systems. Elsewhere across the diaspora, trees are also important to divination and celebration, including contemporary urban African American life.

Calabash in Divination and Celebration

In chapter 2, we devoted much attention to the calabash because it is emblematic of West African healing. It is such an important symbol. The calabash doesn't come from a tree, yet it is forever connected to tree wis-dom by the legend of orisha Osayin, god of the forest. Furthermore, Yoruba followers of *Ife* envi-sion the world as a being divided into two halves, represented by the two halves of a calabash. I also mentioned how it is used as tool, implement, and instrument as well as a story vessel. Now, we look at one of the ways it is used as a tool of divination.

The universe and keys to our existence are held within the shell of the calabash.

Calabash divination is used for communicating with the spirits of a loved one who is absent from the community, whether that loved one is traveling or has passed on. This work is done by a specialist, typically a community healer. Herbs are placed inside the gourd, and a prayer of invocation is chanted to encourage the person or spirit to appear in the water. A libation of palm wine may be used by the diviner to encourage communication from the spirit. If calabash divination is successful, the spirit of the family member imparts news, messages, and inside information through the calabash and water reading concerning the status of the person, which would otherwise be unknown.

> *Oracles are modes of communication that bridge the gap between the domain of spirits and the everyday existence of humans. Words, gestures, sounds, and artifacts remove the separation that conventional ideas of time and space create.*

When a Manding family member is traveling out of Mali, Senegal, Burkino Faso, the Gambia, Guinea, Guinea Bissau, Côte d'Ivoire, and other parts of the middle Niger River Valley in West Africa, their family might use divination to know what is going on with their loved one. If so, the tool of choice is the calabash.[25]

Wood and Plants in the American Nguzo Saba Celebration

In the African diaspora, those of us who observe Kwanzaa have another way of reflecting upon Osayin's calabash of forest medicine and herbal goodness. Kwanzaa, which is Swahili for "First Fruits," is the celebration of a physical and spiritual harvest that puts the sacred wood at the forefront. *Nguzo Saba* (en-goo-zo sah-bah) was specifically designed for people of African descent, which we now realize is every one on the face of the planet. Still, most of its participants are of relatively recent African descent, identifying as black, brown, or multiracial, many of whom live in urban and suburban environments in the United States, where the holiday's originator lives.

Kwanzaa was developed in 1966 by Dr. Ron Karenga, a professor inspired by the great traditions of the classical African kingdoms that are foundational to this book as well, including Nubia and Khemet and the Swaziland Empire, Ashantiland, and Yorubaland. Rather than relying on commercialism like some holidays, Kwanzaa puts spirituality, nature, and ancestors at its core, with the hope of creating stronger black community.

The African words Kwanzaa utilizes are Swahili. In Dr. Karenga's spirit of Kwanzaa, I will use them here for its key features. You don't have to look far into the traditions of Kwanzaa to find the wood. The chalice from which we drink and pour *tambiko* (libations) is usually made from some type of African wood; ours is an unspecified fruitwood. The *kikombe cha umojo* (kee-kom-bay cha oo-moe-jah), unity cup, is made of sacred wood. Placed on *mkeka*, it is used to pour *tambiko* to ancestors

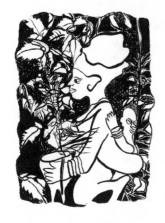

in remembrance, celebration, petition, and praise. The *mkeka* upon which we put our communal displays is made from woven palm leaves. Orisha of the forest Osayin's symbol, the calabash, also figures prominently. I display these, collected from a local farmers market, along with my family and ancestors' photos, because they belong together. When the first day of Kwanzaa rolls around (December 26), I set a few of the most interesting gourds from the group atop the table's *mkeka*. In our personal celebration gourds are a part of *Mazao*, crops, which reflect my spiritual connection to herbalism as mother of the house. Several of the important principles of Kwanzaa are an invitation to engage devotion to the sacred wood:

≫ **Ujamaa** (oo-jah-maah), which is about cooperative economics, fair trade, and supporting your community (stressed throughout this book), is observed December 28. Select a wooden African mask or statue, such as an Ashanti fertility figure (if fertility of any type is desired) from your local African arts and crafts festival or community Afrocentric store. Support African American crafts and artists and shops if you can.

≫ **Kuumba** (ku-oom-bah), the sixth principle, observed December 30, stands for creativity. Create something from your collection from the sacred woods: branches, autumnal pressed leaves or flowers, feathers, bones, etc.

≫ **Imani** (ee-mahn-ee), the seventh principle, observed New Year's Day, is for faith. It is an opportunity to express gratitude to the earth spiritually, through ceremony or ritual.

≫ **Zawidi** (zah-wah-dee), gifts are not obligatory during Kwanzaa; however, on Imani, gifts are sometimes exchanged. Zawidi should be intellectually stimulating; if this is your aim, reach for a kora, balafon, ngoni, and bafako ensemble CD by a reputable group of *Jeli* musicians, an African game like mankala, or a local high school or college spoken word performance.[26]

As you can see, whether we are in the center of the forest, an African village, or an African American neighborhood in the country, suburbs, or city, sacred wood remains vital to our lifestyle, our celebrations, and the maintenance of our community goals. It is up to us to uphold this valuable connection, established and practiced by our people since the beginning of time. The Apagibeti have it right. Let us take their lead, making sure the forest stays open and awake: *"paye awukisi basu,"* the forest saves us.[27]

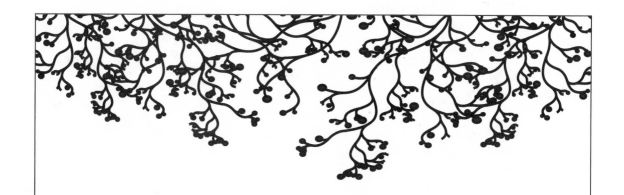

II

Remedies and Rituals
for Daily Life

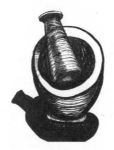

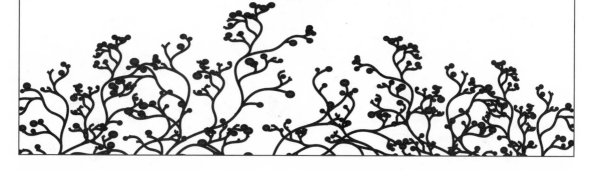

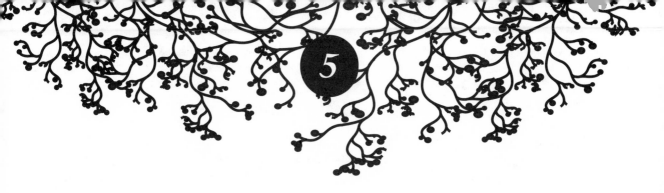

Out Bush

FILTERS, SHIELDS, AND FIELD GUIDES

Lately, my art therapist and I have been working on building filters. Why, you may ask? Because filters trap what's bad, while letting goodness flow through. Think about straining your herbal tea or an energizing cup of Arabica bean coffee, and then think what it would be like instead with herbs or coffee grinds floating about in the cup. Likewise, we want to let the goodness flow into the cup to savor; otherwise we're drinking hot water.

When you start working tree medicine in a holistic sense, making trees a part of your physical or metaphysical neighborhood, you will need filters, and because it is such a potent space, you will need shields and aids of a physical and metaphysical nature. Another important quality is a cool head. There are other features I have been working with during my apprenticeship with a practicing urban shaman here in Chicago—an important one is awareness. Awareness in every world you visit—lower world, middle world, and upper world—is absolutely critical. Even though you may only journey on the astral plane, the sacred wood can be a dangerous place. Likewise, it can be a place where you gain insight, find delightful mosses, delicate ferns, medicinal mushrooms, and other goodies useful in your healing repertoire. You can only find those things if you go in with great spiritual and mental clarity. Intent and focus round out the journey.

What I Learned

I grew up in a rural forest; today I live in an urban one. I learned profound lessons while living in the woods. The lake and the trees that caressed it were my favorite subject matter as a painter; in fact, I think the two drove me to paint. I spent hours watching the currents change, observing the effects of wind and light rain on the water, and listening to sounds coming from iced trees, contrasting them with those moved by summer breezes.

When I went fishing with my father, his awareness was ten times as tuned as mine. He noticed inexplicable things about water and how fish, turtles, eels, and otters moved beneath it. Insects and birds provided additional information for him; fishing birds could reveal the presence of fish, however small, near the surface. Insects comfortable enough to walk or sit upon the water's surface suggested a lack of any fish at upper levels of the lake. In addition, we understood together the landscape of the lake and its surrounding trees and wildlife, watching for changes and new developments. When you're in it, when nature backs up your life, every change is important.

Filtering

I bring up filtering before shielding. The reason is similar to why smudging (submitting a person or thing to fragrant smoke with spiritual or magickal energy) is not a cure-all. Sometimes, smudging is unnecessary or even negative, depending on what kinds of herbs are used. Many smudging herbs are banishing, some are inviting; it is critical to know the trees and herbs wrapped up in your smudge stick, so it can do what you ask. Likewise, if you are entirely shielded, you will not receive; you are blocked and closed.

NORTH AMERICAN INCENSE HERBS

Revered North American healing trees, whose barks and branches are wrapped and tied in the making of smudge sticks or prepared as smolder incense for specific purposes by American healers of African descent and Black Indians, include the following:

Bearberry willow *(S. uva-ursi)*: a prominent American healing tree that is purging and purifying.

Balsam fir *(Abies balsamae)*: native to the northeastern United States and Canada, this sacred tree is used in blessing ceremonies. Fir has pleasing, aromatic quality, considered cleansing and purifying.

Cedar *(Libocedrus descurrens; Juniperus monosperma, Thuja occidentalis)*: called "Desert White Cedar" or "California Incense Cedar," these are preferred smudging cedars. Cedar is burned during prayer, invocation, and house blessings. Cedars ward off illness in the lodge, and in individuals. Cedar works as a purifier and attraction herb when its wood chips are sprinkled over a hot charcoal block or smoldering mesquite.

White Cedar *(Thuja occidentalis)*: burned in purification ceremonies. White cedar is a sacred tree in North America, used primarily in spiritual ceremonies.

Cedarwood *(Cedrus atlantica)*: wood chips can be used as a kindling source for other leaves and branches. Cedarwood is revered for its calming, balancing, ancient wisdom, and is considered a protective plant that aids focus while bringing clarity. The physical aspects are perfect for spring smudging blends. Cedarwood is antiseptic and energizing.

Juniper *(Juniperus communis)*: a revered tree whose needles, berries, and wood are all useful in smudging blends. Juniper is celebrated because it is a tree that is uplifting, protective, purifying, and which boosts confidence and energy levels. Juniper wards off illness and malicious intent.

Mesquite *(Prosopis glandulosa)*: a fragrant wood and ideal charcoal base for burning smoldering herbs during outdoor smudging.

Pine *(Pinus silvestris)*: associated with endurance, perseverance, focus, trust, longevity, community, and stability. American healers celebrate the pine tree for its anti-infectious, antiseptic, tonic, stimulant, and restorative abilities. Pines and other conifers have an important place in early African American burial rites. Their healing medicine has been appreciated from ancient African civilizations to the present.

Piñon: a type of pine needle used in smudging rites, sometimes in place of sweetgrass.

Red Willow *(Salix lasiandra)*: also called osiers or Pacific willow, grows in the Western United States. Willows are prized by many, and used in ceremonial healing.

White Spruce *(Abies alba)*: considered a protective, renewing, grounding, and harmonizing tree that enables us to regain focus and clarity. Other healing properties include antidepressant, antiseptic, and stimulant actions.

Spirits of the Wild

In various African countries, the gifted negotiators, mediating between the spirits of wild and community, are hunters and metalsmiths and in some cases healers, diviners, and warriors. Many tribes, clans, groups, and societies live in very close proximity to wilderness—forest, bush, and savannah—that enforces separation between "wild" and "civilized." Hunters, metalsmiths, healers, diviners, and warriors regularly cross this

> *The world of the forest is a closed, possessive world, hostile to all those who do not understand it.*[1]
> —Dr. Colin M. Turnbull, anthropologist

boundary, helping their communities integrate the power of nature into their daily lives. Generally, these spiritual negotiators recognize and honor various groups of beings residing in wilderness. These beings are somewhat akin to the fairies or pixies of Europe, yet they are more grotesquely misshapen. They also represent inversions of humans, even walking and doing other things backward.

The types of forest spirits ceremonial diviners or masqueraders invoke or repel include:

Abatwa: According to Zulu lore, *abatwa* are very small; in fact, they are capable of shielding themselves with a single blade of grass and sleeping inside anthills. The entire species is said to ride into a village on a single horse. They murder victims with poisoned arrows. It is believed that *abatwa* riding into town on horseback is bad, but if you step on them the repercussions are far worse—this is why keen spiritual awareness in the wood is vital.[2]

Asye usu: Associated with untamed wilderness or bush, these grotesque beings have a demeanor that is erratic and unpredictable, yet some have a desire to help humans, which is arbitrated through divination.[3]

Bori: A densely populated species living in various areas inhabited by or near Hausa people. Dealing with village *bori* is extremely difficult. Forest *bori* are not violent or malicious unless they are harmed or insulted. This might occur by something as seemingly innocent as a fire ember from a campfire becoming airborne and scorching one, in which case *bori* become livid. *Bori* look somewhat like humans but have hoofed feet. They also shape-shift readily, and often appear as snakelike creatures. They enjoy attention. Hausa have elaborate dances, songs, and drummer's rhythms to keep *bori* creatures happy.[4]

Dodo: Possibly the spirit of a dead man wandering the wood, *dodo* is a Ghanaian forest spirit that hangs out with and around Hausa people. This is another shape-shifting species who often take on snake forms. Vicious creatures, *dodo* are ravenously hungry for human flesh and are easily angered. These forest spirits cannot cross running water, so finding a waterfall, brook, stream, or river in their presence would be your key to safety.[5]

PALO MAYOMBE:
FROM THE HEART OF AFRICA TO THE NEW WORLD

While some refer to *Palo Mayombe*, an offshoot of *Santeria*, as its dark cousin, many believe this to be untrue. This path has origins in the Democratic Republic of Congo, from which I have deep ancestry, as do many African Americans who also have Spanish origins. Bantu-speaking slaves are believed to have brought *Palo Mayombe* with them to the United States and some incorporated it into their beliefs.

Palo Mayombe is an earth-based spirituality system. Its primary focus is around the *prenda*s, also called *nganga*s, consecrated ritual cauldrons filled with sticks, stones, roots, bones, and other consecrated and sacred objects. *Prenda* holds the ancestors, and the powerful *nkisi*, which are the deities of *Palo*.[7]

>> **Lucero** is an *nkisi* or deity of the *Palo Mayombe* path that originated in the Democratic Republic of Congo as well. *Lucero* owns openings and crossways such as roads and doors and knows where everything is located—like an ancient navigation GPS but as a deity. He must be handled with extreme care and reverence if you see him. He typically manifests as a young man, naughty but intelligent. He favors rum, cigars, sweets, fish, and possums. His colors are red, black, and white. He can be deadly when petitioned in tight situations. *Lucero* is generally appeased first during *Ebo* (ritual) so he will allow things to go smoothly. His offerings should be taken to the woods.[8]

>> **Ngesh**: Believed to populate the woods, landscapes, and natural water sources of originally Kete lands by the Kuba people of the Democratic Republic of Congo. *Ngesh* are highly regarded as playing an active role in human lives in a favorable way. Diviners consult *ngesh*.[9]

>> **Ope**: Invisible spirits populating forests, mountains, and water sources, *Ope* deliver messages to the Barambo and Poko peoples of the Democratic Republic of Congo. They communicate through dreams and can inflict harm through the manipulation of oracles.[10]

Eloko: A people-eating dwarf living among *Nkundo* people in the rainforests of Zaire, *eloko* live in the hollows of trees in densely forested areas. *Eloko* blend in well with their environment, since they are covered in grass and their clothing is made out of leaves. These dwarves are minute and green, easily mistaken for grass. If that happens, however, they become infuriated. *Eloko* play mesmerizing music, enabling them to overpower and capture their victims. Their favorite instrument is the bell—the bell of death. While the bells are impossible to resist, certain charms and amulets help thwart other *eloko* activities. Only a hunter's magical prowess can dispel angry *eloko.*[6]

BEWARE: DUPPIES OF JAMAICA

In Jamaica resides a spirit, a source of dread, trepidation, and fear, called *duppy.* *Duppies* can be of any ethnicity or race, and of any age—child *duppies* are called pickney. There is a half-cow, half-human *duppy* called a Rolling Calf. The most dangerous is called Coolie Duppy, and it is the spirit of an Indian Obeah man, which are most feared of all. Even though they are spirits, they are said to suck blood from their victims and poison food, especially that of babies and toddlers. They pass from person to person through touch, sometimes from just bumping into a person. The worst contact is if you bump one of them; that can cause stronger illness than contacting someone with a *duppy* inside of them. People make offerings at the buttresses and roots of silk cottonwood trees to placate *duppies*, enticing them either to stay put or to return to their spirit tree home.

Lwa Forest Guides

There is an awe-inspiring tradition of bringing together plant energy with divine, spiritual, and personal energy called vodou. Vodou affirms the relationships between cycles of life, trees of knowledge, and spirit. The vodou vision understands spirits as the intelligence of energy present in humans, nature, and thoughts.

Mysteries can be understood through spirits, goddesses, and gods, known in this path as *lwa.* *Lwa* are intermediaries between Bondye, a very remote, omnipotent god, and humans. The *lwa* were once mortals, and they share some human characteristics, for better or worse, including strength, vision, ego, capriciousness, and fickle

> *In the forest, life appears to be free and easy, happy-go-lucky, with a certain amount of perpetual order as a result. But in fact, beneath all that there is order and reason; reaching everywhere is the firm, controlling hand of the forest itself.*[11]
> —Dr. Colin Turnbull, anthropologist

emotions; they can be demanding and sometimes tricky. Three forest field guides of the vodou pantheon listed below are specific to sacred wood. If you are a student of world mythology, you'll notice that the vodou pantheon embraces universal archetypes of living deities across the planet.

Here is a sampling of important *lwa* to be aware of as you explore the sacred wood:

≫ **Gran Bwa**: This *lwa* helps you connect to ancestral roots or the spiritual home of vodou. Offerings of basins of water, leaves, roots, branches, or flowers are welcomed. A drawing of a "tree of life" is a good conduit to *Gran Bwa*. A tree sapling can be planted on *Gran Bwa*'s behalf. *Gran Bwa* energy exists at each magical point of every tree. Ask *Gran Bwa* to enter the heart, arms, and legs through a ritual dance in the wood.

≫ **Gran Ibo**: Tree talkers, the Divinity Ruth Bass interviewed, and others undiscovered by the outside world were obviously in touch with spirits of the swamp, as are many African American root doctors and treaters (secret doctors) from New Orleans, rural Louisiana, the Southeast, and the Midwest. They would relate well to *Gran Ibo*. Those who find magic and wisdom in the swamp also need to know *Gran Ibo*, lwa of swamps. She understands the language of plants and holds ancient plant knowledge all the way from its roots, because that is where knowledge is held. Everything natural—trees, roots, leaves, pods, flowers, bark, insects, animals, bird, reptiles—all of them find their way through difficulty by attuning to the wisdom hidden in cypress roots. Swamps pulsate with an intelligence capable of nonverbal spiritual commune, if you are open to *Gran Ibo*.

≫ **Olofi**: Seek *Olofi* for balanced *ashe*. Offerings of *kombucha* mushroom tea, roots, artistic symbols, or creative efforts are appreciated. This is the father of *lwa*, patron of earth, an important part of the tripartite aspects of god. *Olofi* represents *ashe* and creativity and can also appear as a pregnant woman, eternally representing Mother Earth—god and goddess as one. [13]

VEVES

Every *lwa* has an elaborate symbolic representation that can be conceived of as a ritual drawing, used to invoke it. *Veves* are drawn on the ground with cornmeal, and they create a pathway between *lwa* and practitioner. Not for the layperson, *veves* are only properly executed by three groups of people: *oungan* (high initiated priest) or *manbo* (high initiated priestess), and *boko*, also called sorcerers. *Boko* can be evil or good. Their work is considered for immediacy, addressing the here and now—they work *veve*, sometimes for less than spiritual ends. [12]

Spirit of the Cloth

You can dress yourself in commanding materials of the forest before you embark on your journey into the sacred wood. The materials you select will determine whether your cloth acts as filter, strengthener, magnet, or shield from negative energy. Looking at known and understood ways of dressing for nature power can be helpful.

Many of us in America like to connect to our African ancestry through cloth. Lots of people reach out for kente cloth, a colorful, readily available cloth. Consider donning these additional cloths when going out into the wood: *adinkra* cloth, for example, is closely associated with the Akan people of Ghana and Côte d'Ivoire. *Adinkra* means "good-bye" to the departed. *Adinkera aduru* is medicine appliquéd in the stamping process of the cloth. Medicines derived from tree barks are applied using iron tool of Ogun (warrior orisha). Designs are created using stamps cut into calabash, which we explored earlier. Originally made and used exclusively for royalty and spiritual leaders, today *adinkra* cloth is important in sacred ceremony and rites of passage. It is worn during festivities, church, weddings, naming ceremonies, and initiations. Every design in the corpus of *adinkra* symbolism depicts something culturally relevant: an iconic proverb, a moralizing tale, an event, a human characteristic, an animal behavior, plant life, or inanimate and man-made objects important to the culture.[14]

Bogolanfini (mud cloth or *bogolan*) fabric from Mali is highly coveted. I feel very powerful when wearing *bogolanfini* in or out of the sacred wood. It is worn by Bamana women during initiation ceremonies and used by hunters in spiritually charged garments. *Bogolanfini* cloth is woven by men and decorated by women with symbolic and readable iconography, capturing Bamana history and lore. The dyes made from soil, tree barks, and leaves demonstrate medicinal knowledge facts, fables, and parables involving people, animals, plants, and deity.[15]

Red Body Paint and Fabric

Red is one of the main emblematic colors of good health. Red is the color of life, representing the life force, power, energy, birth, and renewal. If you want to go into the wood dressed to either give or receive good medicine, wear red. In Ardra, West Africa, red is associated with royalty; elsewhere it is used in menarche and nuptial ceremonies. The three important colors to Yoruba healing medicine are red, called *pupa*, which encompasses reds, yellows, and browns; *funfun*, which is white or colorless; and *dudu*, which we call black.[16] Red is a good color to wear into the forest. Apart from its spiritual significance, it helps set you apart from the greenery of the wood, a good thing during hunting season.

In most African American healing practices, red is an important color. In America, red is used to make flannels, another name for a hoodoo's mojo bag (because the bag itself is often made of soft cloth, preferably flannel). The preference for using red in healing objects and body adornment is attributed to our African heritage, and you can take the lead from the Motherland and wear this power color on your hunt for healing forest medicines.[17]

Head Wraps and Shrouding

People wrap their heads in cloth for religious, spiritual, and style reasons all over the planet. In America we call our head coverings head ties, headkerchiefs, head handkerchiefs, tignons, turbans, and head coverings.[18]* I prefer to have my head wrapped when doing any type of exorcism or spiritual banishing work. This is because I do not want bad spirits in my head or hair. Locs (also called dreadlocks) are believed to be energetic and spiritual conduits. It is important to protect them from collecting negative energy. Some people prefer to cover their head with a wide straw hat or head wrap when going into the forest for many practical or spiritual reasons. One would want to shroud against bugs, particularly ticks, chiggers, mosquitoes, horseflies, spiders, and bees, for example.

In preparation for forest ritual or ceremony, I suggest taking inspiration from our Sudanese and Taureg brothers and sisters, wearing flowing, all-natural, breathable fabric (such as cotton or hemp), long-sleeved, fairly well fitted, light-colored or white robes. White attracts energy of a pure, cleansing nature and it also reflects the sun, so it is cooling. Weather permitting, I will add a natural wool, cotton, or silk shawl to keep energy desired hidden and inside, while opening the shawl to release that which is not. The Taureg of Morocco and environs use turbans as well to conceal their thoughts and protect their identity.[19]

Orishas of Another Kind

The Trinidadian religious group called the Orisha (after the orishas they worship) believe as the Yoruba do that the head, called *ori*, is the seat of the soul.[20] The orishas wear head wraps to *palais* (their holy shrine) but take them off eagerly if an orisha's energy enters the body. Venting is important. Removing the wrap allows

---

*Black and mixed-race women were by law forced to wear tignons in New Orleans and other areas with a high population of mixed-race people (called *gens de couleur* or colored creoles) during the 1800s as a way of distinguishing them from white women.

energy to do its intended work. Once the spirit's energy leaves the head, the head is re-wrapped, helping maintain proper momentum and body temperature. Other cultures also take wraps off during prayer and ritual so they can be in receiving mode.

Conduits of Forest Energy: Mask, Broom, Staff, and Stick

You are immersed in the possibilities of spiritual guides, well versed in some forest spirits to know or avoid, and have been introduced more thoroughly to a variety of African spiritual gear and headdresses for working in the sacred wood, and here are some additional tools to aid your work.

WALKING STICKS

Walking sticks are an important conduit for forest energy. Usually they are created from carefully selected, intriguing (*nyama* and *ashe*-containing) saplings and wood with gnarls and burls, highlighting your walking stick's potentiality. Holding a piece of power-wood in the hand, extending it from your arm to the ground, allows it to become a true energy conduit. This is an important tool of healers in Africa, and there is a very creative tradition of crafting them in the United States, among other areas of the African diaspora. Many self-taught artists working with wood come to work with the walking stick through whittling, a revered rural African American craft.

Often snakes and other symbols are attached to a walking stick, enhancing its inherent power. Nowhere is this easier to see than with the treaters of southwest Louisiana. Here, walking sticks are created for the treater's patients, often with a protective, totemic animal carved on them. Treaters, who view themselves as Holiness healers, not at all connected to a tradition like hoodoo or a religion like vodou (which they consider the "dark side"), call their healing sticks walking canes. To this unique group of African American healers, canes are an amalgamation of craft and power amulet. The best walking cane is one carved by the adept secret doctor who believes in the power of wood and who understands its language—a very African notion.[21] A walking stick is an excellent tool to take on your spiritual exploration, wildcrafting, rite, ceremony, or divination in the sacred wood.

STAFFS

Saints and prophets are often depicted holding a staff. In African culture, staffs are used as medicine of victory and considered a very potent emblem, typically made of all natural materials with additional natural embellishments. Many types of mystical potential are opened up for the person holding a staff.

Nana Bukuu, Mother of Obaluaiye, important Dahomian ancestress of Anagonu deities of the Fon pantheon, was always depicted with a staff.[22] In the womb she had one; when she was born it was embedded in her placenta. After she was born its head curled into a noose shape. It was removed and buried but as she grew so too did the staff. Her staff is called *Ibiriri*, which means roughly "My son found it and brought it back to me," because her son unearthed it after it was buried.[23]

BIRD OF IFA

Osun babalawo, or Bird of Ifa staff, is a distinctive wrought iron staff celebrating or evoking mystical power (*ase*) of Osayin, orisha of herbal medicines and the forest. Commanded by female elders, *awon iya wa*, "our mothers," these staffs possess procreative powers that can be beneficial or destructive. Images of birds are considered to be witnesses to divination, signs of Orunmilla (orisha of wisdom and divination). Perched atop this staff, the bird of Ifa evokes the power to address problems effectively and expediently as only a creature that can touch the heavens can. *Eye Ile* (Bird of House), made of iron, is used as a diviner's staff and by healers to cut and collect plant ingredients for healing or as a weapon against destructive forces. One of the most highly valued possessions of diviners, the staff is placed in front of the diviner's home as a shield.[24]

BROOMS ACROSS CULTURES, TIME, AND SPACE

Nana Bukuu's symbolic image sits atop a baobab tree shrine, represented by a conical piece of earth, wearing raffia, the clothing of spirits. She resembles a large, benevolent whiskbroom. Why would such an important deity as Nana Bukuu be depicted as a broom, of all things? The broom may well be the domestic representative of "spirits of the wild," representing forest and savanna by the very nature of its materials and the ways we learned to use it in Africa. Respect for the broom is an Africanism that we toted in our medicine kit in route to the New World during enslavement. It was a remarkable connection between West Africa and early African American life that apparently survived the transatlantic slave trade.

ORISHA OBALUAIYE'S SHASHARA

A peek at *Ifa* orisha Obaluaiye (because you don't want to leer at this guy too openly) brings greater understanding of the fear and foreboding that brooms provoke. Obaluaiye is a fierce orisha who has power either to create epidemics or to heal them as he sees fit. Obaluaiye's scarlet-clad followers are feared and dreaded. Practitioners believe devotees of Obaluaiye can strike down people who walk around at high noon under the bright sun.

Obaluaiye dispenses epidemic-causing diseases like smallpox when he feels a need to raise the consciousness of society. When the fierce god is angered or appalled by society, he uses his special broom to spread *yamoti* (sesame seeds) across Mother Earth. The horrific tool of Obaluaiye is a magical broom called a *shashara*.

In Benin, Africa, worship of Obaluaiye is called *Sakpata. Sakpata* worshipers also live in Cuba and Brazil. The *shashara* of Cuba are extraordinarily beautiful. Reflecting Dahomean style, these brooms have a special medicated handle covered with symbolic blood-red cloth, heavily embroidered with intricate cowry shell patterns.

ÒJA: AFRICAN BRAZILIAN POWER OBJECT

In Bahia, Brazil, practitioners call the broom *Òja*. In the Dahomean language it is *ha*. Brazilian practitioners of Candomblé elevate *ha* to the level of nobility. The African Brazilian *ha* is a whisk broom transcending utilitarian function, becoming instead an elaborately decorated power object approaching the beauty of finely crafted jewelry. When Obaluaiye appears in Bahian temples, he doesn't carry a club, arrows, or a spear for protection—the only weapon he needs is his *ha*. Obaluaiye's broom is paraded about with flowing movements by his followers; for those aware of its power, this weapon is at once beautiful and terrifying. The motions can suggest both the dispersal of disease-causing sesame seeds and their sweeping away. The Bahian *ha*, also called a *shashara*, is an unusual yet potent royal scepter. It exudes the fierceness of forest energy, yet it is further enhanced by the *ade iko* (all-raffia crown) and complementary *ewu iko* (all-raffia gown) worn by devotees, since they are filled with dual powers of Obaluaiye and spirits of the forest.

BROOM LORE IN THE UNITED STATES

It is only on rare occasions and for specific reasons that spirits of the wilderness are invited into civilized society. These occasions include annual performances, harvest festivals, fertility rites, and (sweeping) purification activities.

Folklore of Adams County, Illinois, lists many methods for healing with broom straw. This book, one volume in Dr. Hyatt's exhaustive research into hoodoo and African American and European American folkloric traditions, customs, and beliefs, cites broom straw as a potent herb that can be used for healing warts. An entire chapter of Hyatt's compendium is devoted to brooms and sweeping. A few entries connect American broom lore back to West Africa, particularly Mende beliefs surrounding the wild, unpredictable quality of brooms as a symbol of the wood. Mende language survived slavery in a creolized form by the Gullah people of the Carolina lowlands, and so did their beliefs regarding brooms.

Several of Hyatt's informants warn that resting or carrying a broom improperly invites injury, pain, or loss. Carrying a foreign broom into the home without following the proper protocol is a sign that death is going to descend on the family. This is probably due to the African notion of the woods and the domestic realm as two distinct conceptual spaces.

Bringing in bits and pieces of the wild, even so straightforward an object as a broom, requires care and consideration, for proper interaction in a spiritual sense brings luck, happiness, and prosperity. Holding a broom under the arm shields against unrest. This most likely carries over from beliefs in the might and power of Obaluaiye and his awe-inspiring, broom-toting devotees. The duality of the broom's uses and the gods, goddesses, *lwa*, and orisha who imbue it with powers makes it an object that can generate luck, domestic bliss, purification, destruction, disease, despair, and, sadly, even death.

Natural Amulets

An amulet exercises control and power for the good of the person who wears it. Intimate contact with the amulet allows the wearer to exert influence over how the amulet's energy is directed. Amulets can be entirely natural but they don't have to be. One of the most common natural amulets used across many cultures is garlic. Hoodoos and rootworkers use mojo bags, amulets containing natural power objects.

An amulet has healing power against illness (in a holistic sense) because the sickness of the wearer is transferred from the person to the object. In this way amulets are used for curing and prevention as well as for protection and power.

MADARIKAN: FORMIDABLE TREE MEDICINE OF THE ONISEGUN

The Yoruba call their herbalists *onisegun* (herbalism is called *egbosi*). Some of the most adept *onisegun* prepare a powerful protective amulet against all manner of psychic, metaphysical, and physical illness called *madarikan*. *Madarikan* are made from different materials, but one of the most highly touted is from the *asorin* tree. This tree has gained its reputation because no other tree grows where it grows—its roots kill any that come too close. The tree's medicine translates as "do not knock your head against mine," demonstrating its intent as the ultimate *ori* shield. The medicine is preventative and protective. Even the most highly skilled *onisegun* barely touch it.[25]

MEDICINE STRING

Worn by the Barambo of Poko of the Democratic Republic of Congo, these are necklaces with impressive power. Plant, animal, and mineral elements are carefully assembled, demonstrating adept environmental awareness and metaphysical focus at once.[26] These medicine strings usually contain a calibrated pattern of elements including seedpods, tree branches, medicinal whistles, tiny gourds, and animal horn—potent symbolic medicines—arranged on the string strategically, evoking prescribed medication called *neo* by the Barambo of Poko.

SHIELDING AGAINST BUGS

I always remember a time I stayed with pagan friends in the Smoky Mountains. I asked for bug repellent and my friends looked at me as though I were speaking a foreign language. It was hot and moist near lots of fresh, running water, so to my way of thinking my request was reasonable. Obviously my friends had developed immunity to the bugs that I lacked, coming from my very different environment. Luckily, during my week of camping in the wood I was not afflicted by bees or mosquitoes. I don't know why.

Not so lucky was my stepmother, who got Lyme disease from tick bites. Practically, you want to shield yourself against bugs, particularly ticks, chiggers, mosquitoes, horseflies, spiders, and bees. Lyme disease can be quite debilitating and it takes a very long time to heal if you can get over it at all. In certain countries malaria is a prevalent disease carried by mosquitoes, and this requires a preventative or prophylactic vaccination. Most experts say products with DEET are most effective for ticks and other biting bugs.

Here are some ways to protect yourself against bugs:

≫ Organic herbal bug repellants include: pennyroyal (which cannot be used by pregnant women), cedarwood, lavender, eucalyptus, and citronella essential oils. Dilute a few drops of these oils in a carrier oil such as grapeseed, almond, peach, or sunflower oil and apply it to your skin.

≫ Lavender makes a good anti-itch treatment if you are bitten by mosquitoes, flies, or gnats. It can be applied neat (directly from bottle) as an organic essential oil.

≫ Mud or clay can be used as a poultice to remove wasp and bee stingers.

≫ Numerous other trees explored later have insecticidal and pesticidal actions.

≫ In the Motherland, a horsehair brush (or one using some other animal hair) is used with a sweeping motion to deflect flying pests.

NEKIRE

Nekire, forest medicine in the form of a whistle, is used by the Barambo to counteract bad spiritual forces. It uses the power of specific trees to yield distinct medicinal properties. Each wood delivers distinct sound possibilities that call on diverse spiritual forces.

NONDUKPALE

Tree medicines with known oracular abilities are harvested to make this amulet. *Nondukpale* provides auguries through physical signs. It gains its power from the wood it is carved from and the plant oils applied to its surface. *Naando* root (*Alchornea floribunda*) is especially popular among Barambo because it brings luck and prosperity.[27]

POD AND HERB AMULETS

I admit I am partial to the devil's pod (*Trapa spp.*) amulet. With its striking, nearly black, shiny, shell-like exterior and freakish resemblance to a bat, devil's pod is foreboding and looks very magical. Devil's pod is also called bat nut, *ling* nut*, and buffalo nut though it is actually a fruit. It was used as a food source in neolithic England. Though it originated in central China, some species have naturalized in North America and Australia.

Everything about *Trapa spp.* suggests it is otherworldly—devil's pod lets us know it is most assuredly not of this earth. I use devil's pod as a protective shield because its biology and mystique make it a force to be reckoned with. Devil's pod is just the right size to tuck inside a mojo bag and is traditionally used in protective mojos. Some use it as an offering to a trickster spirit or dark gods and perhaps it could appease malevolent forest folk. Devil's pod can also be used as a gargoyle to ward off evil.

Devil's shoestring (*Viburnum spp.*) is a natural amulet that grows in woods. The shoestrings are derived from *Viburnum alnifolium* (called hobble bush), *V. opulus* (called European cranberry or cramp bark), and *V. trilobum* (called highbush cranberry) along with others of the species. Devil's shoestring is soaked and pierced with a very strong needle, or wrapped with string and worn around the neck or ankle. Wear this necklace as a protective shield and luck-drawing amulet. Wearing it as an anklet is believed to trip up the devil and bind evil intent, especially that used in hoodoo foot track magic, so this could be especially useful while journeying through the wood. Devil's shoestring can also be placed discreetly in mojo bags.

---

*Ling means "bat" in Chinese.

Job's tears, or prayer seeds (*Coix Lachryma-Jobi*), a species of grass of *maydeae* genus, harken back across the ocean to medicine string. The part of interest suggests seed (and is actually the plant's fruit). The plant grows in marshes and has a place in "secret doctor" medicine for protection and prayer and in hoodoo as a wishing bean.[28] The person making the wish is asked to carry three concealed beads for luck, to throw seven beads in fresh water, or to place a string of beads around a baby's neck to help with teething pain. Job's tears is also called bead plant because it is used to make healing necklaces, "Mary's tears" because it is used to create rosaries, and "tear drops" because of its shape. The plant produces teardrop-shaped, light to dark gray shiny beads with a central hole, just right for making necklaces. The beads are beautiful in their natural state but can also be stained with natural dyes. Seed jewelry has been recorded from early times. In Africa, during the fifth dynasty of Egypt, bodies were found adorned with seed necklaces. Seed necklaces were used against evil on mummified bodies and worn by the living to ward off illness in ancient Khemet.[29] My Yolngu, Pitangara, and Arrente friends in Australia make bead necklaces from bush tucker (wildcrafted foods). My mother frequently wore a powder blue–stained seed bead as a necklace and I now have it. I add organic seed and nut beads to my collection of power amulets when I am accessing energy of the wood in spiritual practice.

Stones as Magical Objects

I like having the energy of Oshun near, so each year I collect river rocks from Thatcher Wood, which has a river running through it. Each spring I mulch my garden with collected river rocks.

ODDUARAS

Be on the lookout after a storm or generally during your walks in the wood for stones called *odduaras*. Supposedly the result of lightning and thunder, *odduaras* are considered to be the property of Chango, orisha of thunder. These stones are used as potent amulets and to create magical spells.

QUARTZ CRYSTAL

Stones of all sorts are considered capable of holding spirits. Minerals and stones play a very active role in African and African American healing traditions. In Daryl Cumber Dance's folkloric compilation *From My People*, she shares collected folklore stating that, to identify a hoodoo or conjurer, see if the person is carrying a beauty pebble (quartz crystal).[30]

THE FAMILY STONE

You can wear any of the following stones or a collection of them around your neck. They can be worn at your ankle to keep your magic close to Mother Earth. Another way to engage the power of stone in the wood is simply to carry your favorite stones in your pockets, medicine bag, mojo bag, or hands. Here are some properties of various stones.

» **Green stones**—Believed to draw prosperity and in some cases health. These include peridot, jade, turquoise, malachite, and aventurine. Emeralds make a wonderful wedding stone.

» **Yellow stones**—Citrine, amber (though amber is a resin, not a stone), and gold topaz are thought to be uplifting, enlightening, empowering, energizing, and attracting because they symbolize the sun.

» **Pink stones**—Rose quartz, tourmaline, and rhondochrosite are stones of the heart, friendship, and attraction.

» **Red stones**—Carnelian, ruby, and garnet are symbolic of life blood; they are cleansers, used for healing, birthing, protection, sexuality, and vitality.

» **Brown stones**—Smoky topaz, certain jaspers, and tiger eye are powerful possessors of animal spirit and magnetism, useful for grounding and centering.

» **Purple stones**—Amethyst and other purple stones are thought of as spiritual stones. They are also used to generate peace or provide blessings.

» **Clear stones**—Crystal or diamonds are sacred stones capable of protection, healing, blessings, and many other purposes.

STONES WITH SPECIAL FEATURES

In addition to the stones listed below, multicolored, striated, and dense stones like onyx, agate, and jaspers absorb negativity.

» **Sodalite**—Improves health, aids sleep, and clarifies sight.

» **Obsidian**—Focuses psychic intent, unhexing energy, and banishing negativity and is used for inner strength.

» **Hematite**—Used for creativity, vitality, and health; it strengthens the heart and blood.

>> **Amethyst**—Used for strength during transformation, weight loss, and overcoming addictions.

>> **Fluorite**—Helps institute "tough love," loving detachment and separations, surviving the incarceration of a loved one; affects the health of bones and teeth.

FOSSILS

Fossils are some of the most sacred gifts of the Great Mother. Fossils are bones of sorts—remnants of ancient life. To charge them, hold them in your hands or put them on your altar. Fossils bring special energy to all of your work. You can also burn incense on top of a fossil.

AMBER

As mentioned previously, amber is not a true rock—it is a resin. With its golden tone and sunny appearance, it is compared to Sun Ra. This resin often has insects trapped inside it, giving us a brief glimpse at ancient life frozen in time. Amber is always warm to touch and is good for warming the sick, thus it enjoys a healthy relationship with healers. An amber necklace is an important protective device when doing clearings and healing work.

CHARGING STONES

Stones seem inert, yet they are actually reservoirs of history, karma, and energy. Each type of stone has its own frequency and unique ability to aid the rootworker. First, though, the rock needs to be charged. There are several ways of charging a rock. Most employ the elements:

1. Bury it in the ground until the stone feels powerful and clear.

2. Place the stone under the sun for three days to one week.

3. Soak the stone in saltwater, rainwater, lightning water, or sweet water.

EXTRAORDINARY PEBBLES AND ROCKS

Malidoma Patrice Some, author of *The Healing Wisdom of Africa*, reports that his people believe that rocks and minerals are reservoirs of memory. Some recommends holding simple rocks and pebbles during memory or remembrance healing rituals.

PETRIFIED WOOD

Petrified wood is ancient, suggestive of the forest's energy, continuity, and inherent power. I use petrified wood as a surface to burn sacred incense and to set up sacred waters.

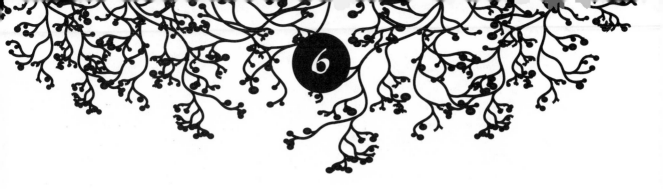

Ways and Means

TOOLS AND TECHNIQUES FOR AFRICA–INSPIRED HERBALISTS

In the next pages, you'll find a list of some of the most useful tools to help you work effectively with tree medicines. Some of these ways may seem very African, whereas others seem more Western. Whatever the geographical source, these tools can enable you to practice African-inspired herbalism safely, effectively, and spiritually.

≫ **Baskets**—Use a basket made from sweetgrass or another handwoven natural material for harvesting and holding freshly gathered nuts, berries, pods, flowers, leaves, bark, moss, and roots. Sweetgrass baskets are made primarily by the Gullah people and sold on Highway 66 and at markets in Charleston, South Carolina, and other low country, seacoast island locations. Some sweetgrass basket co-ops now also make these available online.

≫ **Blender**—Glass or stainless steel pitchers are preferred over plastic because they can be thoroughly cleansed, whereas some residual matter may be retained in plastic, contaminating future blends. Blenders are used for thorough mixing and liquefying a variety of natural ingredients.

≫ **Bottles and jars**—Containers are very important equipment. I like using recycled bottles as much as possible for shampoo and conditioners. Also useful are mouthwash bottles, liquid dish detergent containers, shampoo and conditioner bottles, and lotion, yogurt, and baby food containers. At times, you will want to make special blends as gifts or for sale. There are plenty of specialty container suppliers who carry powder dispensers, sprayer bottles, cologne bottles, flip-top body wash bottles, and decorative jars with screw tops for purposes like this. It's nice, now and again, to use decorative containers for yourself, especially the powder dispensers, since powders are important to African herbalism. There are commercial bottle suppliers listed in the Resources and Organizations section. Remember to sterilize recycled material by boiling plastic containers and cleansing glass bottles with very hot soapy water. Rinse and allow thorough drying before using them. They can also be sterilized in a dishwasher.

≫ **Cauldron**—This doesn't have to be fancy or bought from a specialty shop; a plain cast-iron Dutch oven will do. Dutch ovens made of cast iron are a hallmark of the African American kitchen.

≫ **Charcoal blocks**—Buy charcoal in quantity, as it is the most efficient way to burn loose herbal incense (avoid those that contain saltpeter—it is toxic when burned). Pure bamboo charcoals from Japan are available and make a wholesome alternative.

≫ **Chimenea**—A miniature fireplace, portable and generally kept on the patio, is great for burning incense and is useful in fire rituals if you don't have a fireplace. Chimeneas are growing in popularity and widely available. Sometimes they are simply referred to as patio fireplaces. Look for these at garden centers, home renovation shops, sporting good stores, and specialty shops.

≫ **Coffee bean grinder**—An electric tool with swiveling blades, a coffee bean grinder is a convenient way to grind tough spices and roots, especially compared to its ancestor, the mortar and pestle, which requires hand grinding and lots of elbow grease. Watch out, though—really tough spices and roots need to be ground by hand. They'll break your coffee grinder—trust me, I've gone through quite a few. These are available at coffee shops, home improvement centers, department stores, and discount shops and are indispensable for those with arthritis.

≫ **Double boiler**—An indirect way of heating that prevents waxy mixtures, like ointments and candle wax, from cooking too quickly. A double boiler can be improvised by floating a stainless steel bowl in water in a pot slightly larger than the bowl. This is a great tool to melt and pour soap. Some people use a microwave instead.

≫ **Droppers**—These are essential for dispensing droplets of essential oils, fragrance oils, body fluids, or other precious liquids that you don't want to waste.

≫ **Drying rack**—An implement on which fresh flowers and pods may be hung by their stems and dried. This can also be an attractive way to display and store dried herbs indefinitely.

≫ **Freestanding mixer**—This is a convenient but not essential tool. Use it for whisking and thoroughly blending ingredients while saving your personal energy.

≫ **Food processor**—Even a mini model without all the fancy attachments will do to blend and liquefy ingredients for personal care recipes.

≫ **Funnel set**—Funnels prevent spills and ease the transfer of liquids, oils, and powders from a bowl or pan to a small-necked bottle, referred to here as bottling or decanting.

≫ **Glass storage jars**—Use glass jars for oil infusions and tinctures. Tinted glass spring tops or cork tops work well. And don't forget—sterilize before using.

≫ **Gloves**—Use thick cloth or leather to protect your hands when harvesting berries or encountering other thorny branches. Plastic gloves will keep your hands from contaminating infusions, brews, decoctions, balms, salts, or other handmade herbal blends.

≫ **Grater (Teflon or stainless steel)**—Recommended because these last longer than plastic ones and resist sticking and rusting. Use for shredding beeswax and refining roots.

≫ **Kerchief**—These are made of simple cloth, plain or patterned, and they come in handy for keeping your locs, braids, or any type of hairstyle away from your brews and blends. Some ingredients you work with may be damaging to hair and irritating to the scalp, so it is good to protect yourself while working your tree medicines. It is also important to maintain the highest standard of cleanliness possible so that your herbal blends, brews, and potions are less likely to become contaminated by bacteria, dirt, or oils. (Also see page 67: Head Wraps and Shrouding.)

≫ **Kettle**—Use to boil water for making teas and tisanes, and for infusing delicate herbs.

>> **Measuring spoons**—Stainless steel spoons, with clearly marked measurements etched into the surface, are preferred.

>> **Mixing bowls**—Glass, ceramic, or stainless steel are recommended because they will not become stained from colorants, nor will they harbor bits of left-over ingredients once cleansed properly. Cleanliness is very important; dirty bowls or other equipment will introduce bacteria into your recipes, lessening their longevity and efficacy.

>> **Nonreactive measuring cups**—Both dry and liquid types are useful. Pyrex, tempered glass, and stainless steel work best. Glass and stainless steel measuring cups are easy to clean thoroughly and prevent cross-contamination of ingredients from remnants of herbs and other debris.

>> **Plastic bags**—Use for temporarily containing spices or other dried materials that require airtight storage.

>> **Plastic caps**—Place over the head and hair to trap body heat and encourage the penetration of conditioners and colorants while keeping messy treatments off the neck and clothing.

>> **Pot holders**—Quite a bit of herbal work involves heat, so pot holders to protect your hands from burns are essential when working with infusions, decoctions, and other brews that depend on heat.

SEAT OF THE COMMUNITY: THE MORTAR AND PESTLE

A mortar and pestle is a hand-grinding tool consisting of a bowl and a sticklike grinding tool that can be made of wood, marble, soapstone, or various other materials. In many ways, it is iconic in West and East African village life, and it is an essential tool of both cook and healer. Quite frequently, when African villages are depicted in African stele or other forms of art, the mortar and pestle is figured prominently because the set is considered an indispensable tool for sustenance. Mortars and pestles are used for food preparation, grinding flour from various grains to make bread, and, most important to our discussion here, the mortar and pestle is used to hand grind resins such as frankincense and myrrh, tough spices, barks, roots, berries, grasses, leaves, and flowers. I recommend hand grinding with a mortar and pestle over using a food processor or coffee bean grinder because the process allows the healer to become influenced by the healing spirit energy of the plant. The energy of the plant is released, along with the aromatic oils, as it is being ground, diffusing this energy into the air and imbuing the environment and your soul with force and power.

≫ **Pruning shears**—It is good to have on hand a sharp pair of heavy-duty shears for harvesting woody herbs, plants like roses that have thorns, evergreen branches, and other tough materials found in the forest.

≫ **Scissors**—You will need to have scissors on hand for cutting twine, string, cheesecloth, and leaves.

≫ **Splash-proof apron**—Soapmaking is an important village entrepreneurial endeavor, using oils from African trees such as shea, palm, coconut, and cacao (for cocoa butter). A splash-proof plastic apron is highly recommended protection against the caustic sodium hydroxide used during cold-process soapmaking. Also, consider putting old clothes to work as smocks.

≫ **Stainless steel pans**—Pans with heavy bottoms work best, because they distribute heat evenly and resist burning and overheating. Most important, stainless steel stays inert, preventing contamination and nutrient depletion, which might occur while using aluminum or copper. Make sure you have tight-fitting lids handy as well, as they help retain the medicinal qualities of the volatile oils; otherwise, these precious substances can evaporate. Stainless steel whisks and stirring spoons are recommended for the same reasons.

≫ **Stove or hot plate**—Use for heating, drying, and simmering decoctions, potions, and brews.

≫ **Straining devices**—You can use cheesecloth (muslin) stretched over a preserve or other wide-necked jar, which is secured with a rubber band or twine. I prefer to use a stainless steel sieve.

≫ **Stirring wand**—This is usually made of nonreactive glass or ceramic and is similar to a cocktail stirrer, used to blend perfumes while discouraging cross-contamination.

≫ **Storage bins**—Use to hold dried bark, berries, moss, etc. Dark glass containers with spring tops or stainless steel designs are ideal. Keeping sunlight away from harvested tree parts helps retain their medicinal qualities. Some folks store them in brown paper bags, particularly when they are being dried; this works well only if you don't have moths or other pests that might try to eat the herbs.

≫ **Sun tea jars**—Use glass or plastic jars to brew herbs in sunlight or moonlight.

≫ **Thermometers**—Candy thermometers will work, but a meat probe is my first choice, because it will not break as easily. Thermometers are useful for checking temperatures during the creation of creams, salves, and healing balms, and a thermometer is vital to soapmaking.

≫ **Twine**—Good for tying herbs together at the stems before hanging to dry, and for fixing muslin to jars for straining. Hemp string is an excellent choice for strength and durability.

≫ **Wooden spoons**—With a wooden spoon at the ready, you are bringing the spirit of the wood into your kitchen. Wood in particular will soak in the flavors and memories of many, many potions and elixirs. Wooden spoons bring the power, mystery, and spiritual energy of the forest into your meals. Amass a small collection of these in different sizes and shapes, created from various types of non-endangered wood, for the full effect. Just remember to use safety precautions to protect your wood. For example, they should have as little contact with water as possible. Further, many recipes require stainless steel or nonreactive material, which doesn't include wood. Wood soaks in both good and bad; you don't want essential oils, for example, in contact with your wood.

SPIRIT OF THE WOOD AT THE HEARTH

Using wooden implements instills the spirit of the wood at your hearth. Wooden bowls bring sacred wood into the act of dining, honoring the spiritual and physical connection our people have enjoyed for thousands of years with sacred wood and the great outdoors. Wooden bowls are typically used in America for salads, but in Africa they are also used for main courses and stews. The nice thing is that today you can actually purchase bowls created by various groups of people from African villages. Ten Thousand Villages is a fair-trade store that carries wooden bowls and spoons from several African countries; on a recent trip there, I spotted bowls, forks, and spoons handmade in Kenya.

Releasing Ashe

Once you have a good collection of tools—your means for working forest medicine—the fun is just about to get started, because now you get to consider African ways of working medicines of the sacred wood.

≫ **Agbo** (African infusion method)—A vegetable, fruit (called *aseje*, meaning medicinal food), or herb is infused in water and then squeezed by hand to release the *ashe*. (Yoruba)

> *Divination—a thorough and accurate reading of people, their home environment, and their spiritual and mundane situations—might be just the tool needed for dispensing effective medicine from the sacred wood.*

≫ **Agunmu** (pounded medicine)—Herbal substances, including resins, that are powdered on a grinding stone. (Yoruba)

≫ **Arts**—Dance, drumming, rattles, song sticks, praise songs, performance, masks, and costumes are all used in combination or alone to produce healing effects. (many African societies)

≫ **Ase**—The power of the spoken word and herbal medicine combined. An *onisegun* (herbalist) pulverizes tree medicine and other herbs and puts them on the tip of the tongue before uttering potent incantations.[1] (Yoruba)

≫ **Ashe**—*Ashe* is such a powerful and mysterious word that it really is untranslatable.[2] It is partly a spiritual command, and it is very desirable during divination because it enables smoother contact with ancestors and spirits. I use this word frequently in the manner of an herbalist to describe the healing elixir present in the liquid essence of a tree, plant, root, flower, bud, berry, or leaf. (Yoruba)

≫ **Decoction**—A detoction is made by extracting medicines from tougher parts of the plant, including the roots, bark, or berries. Decoction is accomplished by simmering the tough parts of the tree in a covered pan of water, over medium-low heat, for from half an hour to five hours, depending on the degree of toughness. Once this process is complete, *ashe* is readily available for healing work in the brew, which is formally called a decoction but can be called a potion or by another name. (mainly Western)

≫ **Divination**—As I've said, tree medicine isn't simply harvested and worked like biomedicine; it has recognized metaphysical and spiritual content. Divination plays a role in determining what medicine to use, how much, and for which individual. (cross-cultural)

≫ *Etu* (burnt medicine)—Slowly charring ingredients in a pot, which is typically made of cast iron or another heavy metal. The *etu* is then consumed as is or used in a body rub. *Etu* has a role in soapmaking and may describe plants that have yielded potash, as well. (Yoruba)

≫ *Igbere*—Yoruban technique of injecting medicine in the manner of a vaccination, subcutaneously.

≫ **Infusion**—Can be either water-based or oil-based. Water-based infusions are teas containing *ashe*, also called tisanes or brews. Infusions are made by extracting the volatile oils of a plant by pouring boiling distilled water over the herb and keeping it covered for thirty minutes to one hour. Heating them in water for a longer time on a very low temperature on the stovetop will infuse tougher herbs. The pot should be tightly covered to retain the healing medicine rather than allowing it to escape into the air. (cross-cultural; mainly Western, more likely called tea or used as bath in Africa and African diaspora)

≫ *Iwa rere* and *Iwa pele*—Level-headed energy; mind, body, and spirit in balance; tranquility, coolness; an even-handed temperament when attempting divination, conjuration, or healing using tree medicines; important and helpful. (Yoruba)

≫ *Kia*—A transcendent state that allows spirits to move through the healer, usually brought about through dance and movement. (!Kung/South African)

≫ **Maceration**—A method of releasing the volatile oils and delicate scents of buds and flowers. To macerate buds, mash them up in a mortar with a pestle, or pulse for thirty seconds in a mini food processor. (cross-cultural; started in Khemet)

≫ **Magical spirit hand**—Often, the hand opposite from the dominant hand is used in the preparation and consumption of magical or spiritual medicines. This hand is typically the left hand, considered the magical hand, as many people are right-handed. If you are left-handed, switch to your right hand if using this technique, because that would be the special hand for you, the one you seldom use in mundane activity. (Africa and African diaspora)

≫ *Mampiboaka tromba*—A method of calling out to spirit directly. Through *mampiboaka tromba*, you call out to good or bad spirits to state the intentions behind bringing mental, physical, or metaphysical illness, and request identification of what type of spirit is involved, under whose agency it works, what it wants, how it should be addressed, and what it requires to leave. This technique may include praise songs.[3] Once the *tromba* (royal ancestor spirit) says its name, it is no longer considered powerful. This East African technique is strikingly similar to the Yoruban and African American technique of directly addressing illness caused by spirits. (Malagasy/Sakalava people)

» *Mafutas*—This is a practice using fat, with or without trees and herbs, from a wide variety of animals, reptiles, and insects, including the bull, baboon, eagle, puff adder, porcupine, monkey, wildebeest, iguana, hippopotamus, giraffe, and chameleon, for their medicinal value. (Zulu/South Africa) The animal is selected for magical, spiritual, and mythological significance as well as for the vitamins, minerals, and enzymes it contains.[4] It is interesting to note that, in early African American culture, the first thing put into a baby's mouth for luck and longevity was a piece of fat.

» **Oil-based infusion**—You can extract the volatile oils from herbs by putting herbal materials into a sterilized (dry) container. Fill the jar to the top with loosely packed flowers, moss, or tender leaves. Pour on the preferred oil (such as olive, sunflower, sweet almond, or safflower oil) to cover. Cover the jar tightly. Let these infuse six to eight weeks. Strain to remove the herbs. An excellent combination is a (tree medicine) sweet almond oil and (herbal) calendula flower petals infusion. This works great applied directly on sensitive skin for burns, rashes, and irritation. (started in Khemet/now used in the Americas and elsewhere)

» *Olugbohun*—An amulet with special *ase*, prepared in the horn of a bull and partially wrapped in symbolic cloth.[5] (Yoruba)

» *Oruka*—An herbal medicine ring; medicine that is worn externally to affect the holistic health of the patient. (Yoruba)

» **Patience**—It should go without saying, but many feel it is OK to handle tree medicines forcefully, but in this process the medicine loses the potentiality of the plant to heal. Patience is critical. Whatever means are used in the healing process, it generally takes time and lots of it. (universal)

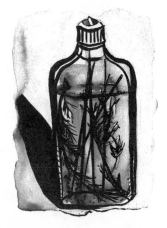

» **Praise**—Each tree has a protocol for planting, growing, harvesting, and using. Even though you may be uninitiated, it is vital to be thankful to the tree for giving its life force in an effort to assist your healing work. (African diaspora)

≫ **Prayer**—Generally, thanks are given at the time of planting, during the growing process, harvesting, and when processing tree medicines. This can take the form of a chant, praise song, or prayer that incorporates your faith. (universal)

≫ **Tincture**—The extraction of healing medicines from herbs, created by using hundred-proof alcohol such as vodka, grain alcohol, or rum. The concentration of volatile oils is greater in tinctures than through infusion or decoction. Fill a sterilized jar to the top with loosely packed herbal material. Be sure to use an alcohol like vodka (do not use rubbing alcohol; it is too harsh and it smells so strong that it will overpower any attempts to scent it). Cover the herbs with the alcohol and cover tightly. Place the jar on a sunny windowsill and swirl it gently every day for four to six weeks; strain off the herbal material and pour the tincture into a sterilized tinted bottle. (Americas and Caribbean)

≫ **Toddy**—Since the time of the ancient African civilizations of Axum, Kush, Nubia, and Khemet, African healers have combined herbal infusions with wine or other alcoholic beverages. (cross-cultural, today mostly Jamaica)

Spirit Works Within the Roots

Knowing proper harvesting, drying, handling, and extracting techniques is essential to African herbalism, but technique is by no means the last word. The term *workin' roots*, as in rootworker, means you need to work, not just use. Incorporate affirmations, incantations, prayers, and even numerology or astrology as well as meditation in the process of working tree medicines to access their full spirit energy.

Speaking directly to the pot, fire, candle, and tree is also essential. I have demonstrated that this is done throughout Africa and the African diaspora. It is important to address each element or aspect of nature with the assertion that it is alive. Organic objects are replete with potentiality and healing *ashe*, so they have a universal energy force within, connecting us all like an umbilical cord. To simply *use* herbs, flowers, stones, bones, fire, or water without paying homage to their life force insults the spirits. In Haiti, for example, spirits mount humans, helping them carry out healing work. Healers influenced by various *lwa* (spirits) fall into a trancelike state; some dance during healings, while others sing or chant. In the United States, many African American healers commence their work with prayers, psalms, or songs. Bringing together spirituality with healing work is an exciting experience, and it is also a distinctive aspect of African herbal healing. Opening the door to the metaphysical adds even more possibilities.

Boiling Energy

In Western herbalism, we advise against boiling any type of herbal material, preferring to infuse or decoct through simmering instead. West Africans like to maintain an evenness that is sometimes described as cool and balanced, or *Iwa rere* and *Iwa pele* or *deu* by South Africa's !Kung. !Kung practice a fascinating healing technique where they build *num*, healing energy.[6] The practice involves a great deal of dancing. A newer, contemporary dance that has been evolving since the 1970s is the Dance of the Trees. The more traditional dance is the Giraffe Dance. It can involve as many as eighty dancers and thirty singers of all sizes, shapes, sexes, and ages from the community.

These dances can last for hours, all through the day or night. The desired state is one of ecstasy called *kia*, which allows spirit to move through the healer. When the energy level reaches a climactic height, it is a tumultuous experience called boiling energy.[7] When *num* (healing energy) builds and spills over, boiling energy can be transmitted to others during communal healing activity, typically through Tree Dance or Giraffe Dance. Afterward, the healer and group are given time to cool down, called *Hxobo*, to release the intensity of spiritual contact and return to mundane activities.[8] This activity of southeast Africa has correlations to West African and central African divination practices as well as practices of the Caribbean and Americas, particularly the African American churchgoer's experience of "getting happy." "Getting happy" happens when the spirit of God or Jesus Christ moves through the body of a parishioner, sparking a dance or shuffle of ecstasy. This happened quite frequently with my mother at church. At first I found it a major embarrassment, but it became infectious. In Haiti's vodou practice, a similar experience occurs when the priest or priestess is "mounted" by *lwa* (spirits).

Mindful Harvest

Clearly there is a spiritual side to healing, very strong in African people, and often it mimics or utilizes forest energy. Crossing spirituality with tree medicines involves age-old techniques that approach metaphysics. There is also a practical side, involving the

> *Quiet thoughts that blossom in a fertile mental environment inside a balanced mind might be your key to effective healing.*

extraction and processing of tree medicines closer to a biomedical approach. In a nuts-and-bolts manner, a good herbalist attempting to establish an Africa-inspired herbal practice hones her or his skills as a dancer, musician, singer, herb doctor, and rootworker. The closer these facets can be brought together, to the point when they begin to effortlessly mesh, the more efficacy is obtained in this type of healing. Be alert and aware of wider aspects of the forest than just trees. Obviously omens, signs, and symbols of things living in and near the wood, as discussed in the last chapter, should be considered. Proper protocol while harvesting medicines of the forest should always be developed holistically, considering the overall environment impact, tree and community health, and the most wholesome way of extracting the medicines.

I recommend following a basic African tenet—coolness. Decide how to dress appropriately for obtaining and maintaining power. Consider the animal omens, shield yourself, and use filtering techniques. Go out bush for gathering with a clear head, balanced and well rested, preferably after practicing twenty minutes or so of simple yoga asanas or hatha yoga meditation. Grab your favorite palm or sweetgrass basket and proceed.

TIPS FOR HARVESTING LEAVES

Look for leaves of a consistent green color, without brown or yellow spots. Harvest mid-morning, after any dew has evaporated. Gather leaves before the plant begins to flower. For plants such as basil or oregano with long growing seasons, pinch back the tops to prevent flowering (flowering takes energy away from the growth of the plant). Keep herbs separated by type, and tie their stems together loosely in a bundle with twine or hemp string. Until you are very familiar with all the tree medicines on your route, it is best to label bundles and date them as well. Hang them up to dry immediately after harvesting to prevent mildew or deterioration.

Hang herb bundles stem-up in an area with good circulation, away from direct sunlight. The ideal temperature for the first day is ninety degrees, followed by seventy-five to eighty degrees the rest of the time. Most herbal bundles will dry in two to three weeks. Petals and leaves should feel light, crisp, and paperlike. If there are small buds or tiny leaves, which may fall off during drying time, create a roomy muslin bag to encase the flowers and leaves. Tie it loosely with twine or hemp string at the stems. This is particularly important with seed-dropping plants. When herbs are completely dry, store the whole leaves and stem away from direct sunlight, in dark glass or stainless steel airtight containers.

HARVESTING FLOWERS

Select healthy flowers in early afternoon, during dry weather conditions. Flowers are extremely delicate. Take extra care not to bruise the petals. Try not to touch them.

Cut the blossoms from the stems and allow the flowers to drop into your basket. It's best to dry smaller, more delicate flowers such as lavender and chamomile whole. Hang them upside down, tied with twine over a muslin cloth or large bowl, or wrap loosely with muslin to retain the dried buds.

Use fresh flowers whenever possible. You may also freeze flowers in an ice cube tray filled with spring water.

HARVESTING SEEDS

Collect seeds on warm, dry days. Seeds need to dry in a warm, airy environment. Make provisions to catch quickly drying seeds by placing a bowl or box underneath hanging plants.

HARVESTING BARK

Bark peels most easily on damp days. Choose a young tree or bush, if possible, one that has already been pruned, cut, or taken down naturally by wind or stormy conditions, to prevent causing damage or even death to the tree. Stripping too much bark from a tree will kill it. A thoughtful approach to Mother Nature's gifts is essential. Bark may harbor insects or undesired lichen, so wash it and allow it to dry flat on waxed paper, in a location that is well ventilated and away from direct sunlight.

HARVESTING ROOTS

Roots are ready for collecting after autumn harvest. Dig up roots after their plant has begun to wither and die. Extract the root while trying not to bruise it. Like bark, roots need to be cleaned and dried before use; they also require ethical harvesting. Cut roots into small sections, and dry in an oven set between 120 to 140 degrees. Turn and check them regularly. Roots should feel light and airy, like sawdust, when fully dried.

HARVESTING BERRIES, FERNS, AND MOSS

Use the same procedure as for bark, but remember that berries and fruits take a long time to dry, about twice as long as leaves. Flowers, ferns, and mosses should be dry without dew, so waiting a few hours into the morning is best. Obviously, do not harvest during a storm, since this book is focused around tree medicines, unless your work includes elemental magick.

HARVEST ETHICALLY

Be especially careful about barks and roots; some plants are overharvested and face extinction. To avoid making a negative environmental impact, remain aware of the status of the trees you seek to work with. For example, is the tree endangered or fragile? If so, seek alternatives.

While this isn't usually a huge problem when buying tree products from African sources as most are wildcrafted, if they aren't from Africa, ask: How they are grown? Are they organic or wildcrafted? It matters. Wildcrafted or organic materials are the most ethical and safest ingredients to use in poultices, baths, facials, massage oils, personal care products, and consumables.

When purchasing your tree seeds, pods, nuts, oils, essential oils, fixed oil, barks, and so on, ask yourself:

≫ Are the prices fair, without excessive markups? Do some research and price comparisons.

≫ Is what you want usually in stock, available without delays?

≫ Is the source convenient and practical for you?

≫ Is a knowledgeable person available to answer your questions?

≫ Are the products fresh? Always look for freshness, even with dried medicines and spices (look for bright color, no mold or mildew, strong scent), and check expiration dates.

≫ Key: Does this company have fair-trade projects with African, Caribbean, or American (North or South) companies? They should, if that is where the products are grown. This affects the spiritual efficacy of your medicines. Does this company give back to the community from which it harvests?

To summarize: Yes, there are tools, equipment, and methods, what I refer to as ways and means, but there is also spirit—the spirit of nature, power words, performance arts, ancestor spirits, and the spirit within your *self*. Be sure to remain attentive to your intuition as you work all the tree medicines available in the sacred wood, because often intuition is the way spirit communicates and assists with your healing practice.

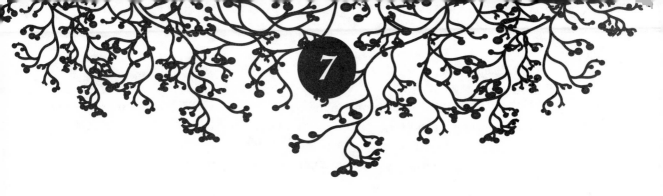

Seeds, Nuts, Pods, and Oils

How does one categorize seeds, fruit, nuts, and pods? I divide them into conceptual spaces rather than botanical allotments, prying the nut with difficulty from the fruit, to give these chapters some breathing room. My aim is to examine the plant parts, focusing on their impact on holistic health in Africa and our diaspora. As you shall see, seeds, pods, and nuts have been significant food sources and economic components for African people for thousands of years and have also acted as our health insurance policy. These plant parts have played an important role in community wellness, with a leading role in integrative medicine. We use nuts, pods, and seeds for protection amulets, adornment, divination, ritual, and ceremony. We use them to dress wounds and prepare for weddings, and we use them after giving birth, and much more.

We had an orchard in our family through my Aunt Ann. The Brockinboughs, who had lived in Salem County and surrounding environs far longer than I had, were influential in our move to the area. Aunt Ann's sister's family, the Drains, had a cozy family nut and fruit orchard just outside

Woodstown. Like many people in the area, they had an off-the-road fruit stand, and they made pies and gave bushels away to family and friends—lucky us! Each year, energy permitting for climbing ladders and such, we could have hazelnuts, cherries, and apples for canning, baking, and other wholesome blends.

At the Boone Plantation outside Charleston, South Carolina, pecans are one of the chief crops, even today. In Charleston, we ate wonderful praline pie baked by Gullah people in Mt. Prospect. Elsewhere in that area of the southeast, we enjoyed peanut brittle and boiled nuts. Of course, peanuts are legumes; we call them nuts, but they are an important source of protein enslaved Africans brought to the United States. African American inventor George Washington Carver invented peanut butter, which is similar to West African groundnut butter.

Seed: fertilized, matured ovule of a flowering plant, containing an embryo of rudimentary plant; the propagative part of a plant, preserved for growing a new crop.

Nuts don't have to be sweetened to taste good. Actually, in their plain state their phytonutrients are most intact and available. Plain peanut butter is best used in peanut butter bread, sandwich snacks, or stews. Plain nuts, ground or not, contain healthy oils. Some have shells that produce medicinal teas and natural dyes, for example the black walnut, which is in the same aromatic tree family as the pecan. Walnuts make an astringent good for treating wounds, and the shells yield a superb dye for brunette hair and for virgin wool for knitting. Walnut oil is light enough to use in salads, and it makes outstanding hair oil, though it is somewhat pricy as the demand for it relative to other nut oils is low.

Bean: edible, nutritious seed of plants from the legume family; plant producing beans as seeds; pod of this type of plant; any bean-like seed or plant.

Pod: usually elongated, two-valved seed vessel; can be of the pea or bean; the dehiscent (open) fruit of a leguminous plant; dried, several seeded, dehiscent fruit or seedpod.

Some of the most important trees in the world for food products and beauty preparations created from nuts, pods, kernels, oils, and butters originate with Africa and the African diaspora. I'm willing to bet that you have some of these agroforestry products in your home right now. These oils and butters are also economically vital to many rural African communities; our lives would be tough without them. I'm talking about:

>> Palm trees, which yield palm kernel oil and coconut oil, among others. Palm and coconut oil are in most packaged and many bakery-produced baked goods, beauty products, natural soaps, and more.

>> Cacao trees, from which we get cocoa, chocolate, and cocoa butter.

>> Shea trees, from which shea butter is made by African women and children.

>> Chocolate itself usually contains both shea butter and cocoa butter.

>> And spices—our world would be bland without them—some of which are actually seed kernels that also produce oils and butters.

There are also delightful North African oils, such as sweet almond, moringa, and balanites. Some you may not have heard of but will become more familiar with are:

>> Jatropha oil, a biodiesel so pure that it doesn't need to be refined to fuel a diesel tractor. It brings much needed income to rural communities, facilitating soapmaking cheaply.

>> Mongono nut is in large part a sustenance food for a large group of South Africans.

>> Foraha oil has more remedies and applications than you can shake a stick at.

Some of the trees featured in this chapter are quickly approaching the status of "miracle oils." What I've decided to do here is describe the trees, their origins, local folk and contemporary/global uses where applicable, and what each of these wonderful African trees can do for you.

Balanities

Balanities (*Balanities Aegyptiaca*), called *heglig* in modern Egyptian Arabic, are trees with thorns. They are found in most arid or semiarid to sub-humid tropical savannahs and many hot, dry areas along waterways and forests. The tree is native to the Sudano-Sahelian zone, Israel, Palestine, and Jordan. Balanities trees are flexible, but they cannot tolerate prolonged flooding.[1]

QUALITIES AND USES

≫ The balanities seed consists of 30 to 40 percent oil. The plant is a useful soap substitute because of its high saponin content.

≫ Locally, balanities oil is useful in treating sore throat, colic, mental diseases, epilepsy, and toothache, and it serves as a laxative.[2]

≫ Balanities oil may be useful applied as a hot oil treatment to the scalp and ends of hair for those with overprocessed, chemically treated hair.

≫ Analgesic qualities lend balanities oil the ability to reduce the sensation of pain, making the oil useful, when warmed, as a massage treatment.

≫ Astringent balanities oil should be combined with other emollient ingredients like avocado, jojoba, or castor oil when used on dry skin or hair.

Moringa Oil

Also called the drumstick tree, in modern Egpytian Arabic *ban* or *jasar*, and horse-radish tree and oil bean tree in Ghana, moringa oil (*Moringa stenopetala, M. Oleifera M. pterygosperma; M. aptera*) comes from Egypt, the Sudan, and the Arabian penin-sula. M. pterygosperma is indigenous to Egypt and still grows there. It is favored for cosmetics and cooking.[3] Moringa has a long history, recorded in Egyptian medical papyri, as a woman's pregnant belly rub, called *ben*. Pharaohs also used it as a treat-ment for gum disease that included moringa, gum acacia, figs, water, ochre, and four other ancient plants.[4] Moringa contains 73 percent oleic acid and other nutrients. Today, moringa continues to be used in skincare products, in perfume and soap, and as a lamp fuel. This oil makes a delightful vehicle for essential oils, making it useful to massage therapists and practitioners of aromatherapy.

The roots are acrid, digestive, antihelmetic, constipating, anodyne, bitter alexi-pharmic, stimulant, and vesicant. Moringa is useful in inflammation, fever, cough, cold, bronchitis, pectoral diseases, epilepsy, and hysteria. The leaves are used to treat scurvy and vitiated conditions. The seeds are an acrid bitter, useful in neuralgia, inflammation, and intermittent fevers.

Sweet Almond

The almond tree (*Amygdalus communis* Linn.) is a spiny tree growing in warmer climes. Native to North Africa and western Asia, it now also grows in many other temperate countries. The tree is moderately sized, from twenty to thirty feet high, with broadly spread branches and lance-shaped leaves with finely serrated edges. *Amygdalus communis* var. *dulcis*, which yields sweet almonds, produces pink flowers in early March in the United States. A member of the family *Rosaceae*, sweet almond is related to the rose, plum, cherry, and peach.

KEY FEATURES OF SWEET ALMOND OIL

Sweet almond oil is almost clear, though it can appear faintly yellow. It is a nearly odorless liquid with a slight nutty taste and a lighter feel than olive oil. It is a valuable lubricant for fixing watches. It is a fine ingredient for handmade soapmaking and the formulation of cosmetics. It softens and works wonders on dry winter skin, parched lips, and calloused hands. It has been used historically to alleviate pain as a massage oil and to remove age spots, pimples, and wrinkles. I hold this oil in very high regard, finding a little of it to go a long way. I appreciate its lack of odor, preferring to add my own essential oils for scent and to accentuate its therapeutic action. It does not leave you smelling like food or nuts as can be the case with stronger scented oils such as olive oil.

BENEFITS OF ALMOND OIL

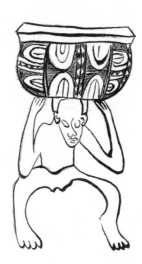

> Rich in protein

> Contains mineral salts

> Good source of vitamins A and B

> Sight tonic

> Antiaging (contains vitamin E)

> Alleviates constipation

> Calms internal inflammations

> Emollient

> Used to relieve itchy dry skin

> Gentle enough for hypoallergic skin and babies

Jatropha

Jatropha (*Jatropha curcus L.*), family *Eurphorbiacea*, was introduced to Africa by the Portuguese and grows very well there. It grows on the Cape Verde Islands and has been naturalized in the West Indies, growing in Jamaica and Brazil. It is well suited to arid and semiarid conditions. Most jatropha trees thrive in areas with seasonal dry weather, like grassland and savanna and thorny forests. It is tenacious and drought resistant, growing well in poor soil. It can produce seeds for fifty years. Jatropha is a small tree that can grow from eight to fifteen feet.

PROPERTIES AND USES

Jatropha oil is rich in glycerin, making it useful in various hair care, scalp, and skin treatments. In 1999, the Alternative Resource for Income (ARI) project successfully mobilized women to produce handmade soaps from jatropha oil to fight skin ailments such as eczema, acne, rashes, psoriasis, and fungus.[5] The latex from the trunk contains the alkaloid jatrophine, which is showing some promise as an antioxidant. In Surinamese traditional medicine, jatropha leaves are used as a bellyache treatment for children. The boiled leaves are used as a dentifrice for gingivitis and throat ailments. The leaves are also used to treat urinary blockages, constipation, and backache as well as other areas that become inflamed. Rubefacient (warming) properties are contained within the leaves, making them suitable for poultices, salves, balms, or soak treatments for rheumatism and for eruptions like boils and piles.

> ### TREES AS RENEWABLE ENERGY SOURCES
>
> Biomass energy is produced from plants and animal matter. Biodiesel is fuel made from a renewable source such as plants. Jatropha, being an easy tree to grow and whose kernel is 50 percent oil, is being used in different countries as fuel for diesel engines.

The seeds are emetic, causing drastic cathartic effects, accompanied by burning feces, burning stomach, and other serious symptoms. Their use should be avoided. The seeds have a 50 percent oil content.

Jatropha is used to treat cancer, piles, snakebites, paralysis, and dropsy. The tree contains constituents capable of attacking infections of the scalp that normally deter hair growth. It is considered an invasive weed, but obviously it is useful for multiple purposes. Jatropha is being used for an ecofriendly biodiesel fuel that burns without smoke, powering simple diesel engines without the need for refinement.[6]

Jatropha used as a biodiesel has the following attributes:

≫ Less polluting than petroleum (a nonrenewable energy)

≫ Lower emissions of carbon dioxide, sulfur dioxide, particulate carbon monoxide, airborne toxins, and unburned hydrocarbons

≫ Clear, smoke-free flame

In addition, it:

≫ Makes an organic fertilizer

≫ Shows promise as an insecticide

Mongono

Mongono (*Ricinodendron rautanenil*)is called *mungongoma* by the Shona people, *mongongo* or *mugonga* by the Tswana, and *xa* by the !Kung. Like Jatropha, mongono is a member of the Euphorbia family. It is a large, spreading tree that grows 15 to 120 meters tall. It produces yellowish flowers on slender, loose sprays. Mongono is distributed widely throughout southern Africa, growing well in northern Namibia, northern Botswana, southwest Zambia, western Zimbabwe, Malawi, and eastern Mozambique.

The flesh of the mongono fruit, which can be red or green, can be eaten fresh or dried. Fresh, it is spongy and tastes sweet, like a date. When it is dried the fruit can be edible up to eight months. The skin makes up 10 percent of the fruit, the flesh 20 percent, and the nutlike seed 70 percent. The seed's outer shell is hard and porous. Elephants eat them, and some people find them easier to consume after they are passed through the elephant.

The creamy yellow nutmeat is oily and nutritious. It is rich in polyunsaturated fats, almost all lineoleic.

INDIGENOUS USES

Indigenous southern Africans who still hunt and gather, in Namibia for example, eat one to three hundred of the fruits per day. Some people report eating up to 950 per year. Bantu, Khoi, and San people use the fruits to make various dishes, including a modern innovation of tasty reddish porridge, similar in consistency and taste to applesauce. Mongono is the staple diet of the San of northern Botswana and Namibia, where it has been consumed by the San people for at least seven thousand years. It is also a key food source for the !Kung people. Its popularity stems from its flavor.

High vitamin E content stabilizes the Mongongo nut, keeping it from perishing quickly. The oils from the nuts are used as a body rub, to clean and moisten the skin. The nuts are also used as divination tools, with the outer shells serving as divination bones.

Nutmeg and Mace

More familiar for many readers than jatropha or mongongo are the spices nutmeg and mace. In fact, these old-time spices are so familiar that we barely think about what they are or where they come from. *Myristica fragans*, their source, is an evergreen tree with aromatic leaves, tiny yellow flowers, and fruits that split, revealing a sweet-yet-spicy seed kernel called nutmeg. The seed looks for all intents and purposes like a nut, just about the size and shape of a very small walnut, though smoother and darker.

Mace is the arillus, a leathery coating between the stone and pulp of the fruit, usually an amber-orange brown color once dried and sold in trade. It is purplish red when first harvested. Nutmeg grows from twenty-five to thirty feet high in coastal, humid tropics.[7]

Myristica fragrans originated in the Moluccas, Indonesia, but is also grown in Grenada. Just about all of America's nutmeg and mace comes from Grenada, a very small Caribbean nation located between the Caribbean and the Atlantic Ocean, north of Trinidad and Tobago. The population is almost entirely African descended: 82 percent identified as black and 13 percent biracial; the rest are native Caribbean groups. Over two thousand tons of nutmeg and mace were exported from Grenada in 1994, making it one of their top exports.[8] A smaller crop comes to the United States from St. Vincent, also a Caribbean Island.

USES

≫ Nutmeg and mace can be used as spices, preferably when they are whole and top grade (see sidebar).

≫ Nutmeg and mace have a warming, aromatic, resinous taste; they are typically grated in small enough amounts to use at once, or they lose flavor.

≫ This spice blend figures prominently in winter holiday seasonal foods such as eggnog, mulling spices, gingerbread, custard pies, and sweet potato pie.

≫ Nutmeg is used for quiche and white potato pie, and for seasoning meat products.

≫ Nutmeg's constituent *myristicin* is a hallucinogen.

≫ Used in perfumery, especially men's cologne.

≫ The pharmaceutical industry uses nutmeg and mace for its many medicinal properties.

≫ Lesser grades are made into essential oils, oleoresin, and butters for cosmetics.

≫ Nutmeg eases digestion, nausea, and flatulence.

≫ Used as an aphrodisiac, it also increases the intoxicating effect of alcoholic beverages.[9]

≫ Used in magickal herbalism as a scent and scent fixative, and in potpourri and incense.

WHEN NUTMEG AND MACE GO BWP

You might not think often about spices getting old or going stale, but you should. Like anything else in your holistic kitchen, the spices should be kept whole and fresh. I typically buy my nutmegs with mace intact, whole from a spice dealer, and I do the same with cinnamon, juniper berry, allspice, and peppercorns—grinding them all myself as needed. This adds incredible flavor and sizzle to recipes, making me feel like a gourmet, though I am not. Nutmeg and mace are perfect for adding to potions, mojo bags, and handmade incense and potpourri because they can be imbued with *ase* and *ashe* as you work.

With nutmeg and mace, you want to be particularly careful about buying whole and fresh, for health reasons as well as taste. BWP (broken, wormy, and punky; from Indonesia) or "floats" and "defectives," as they are called when from Grenada and St. Vincent, carry mold, and too much of the toxic chemicals aflatoxines to be safe for consumption, but some unscrupulous spice companies sell them ground into spices.[10] I grind my nutmeg in a mortar and pestle, releasing the mace gently by hand, or I use an electric coffee bean grinder to work more quickly. Two companies with Internet outlets selling fresh nutmeg and mace are Penzey's Spices and San Francisco Herb and Natural Food Company.

Kweme

Kweme (Telfairea pedata), also called oyster nut, comes from Tanzania. It also grows as a perennial in central and east Africa. It is native to Mozambique and Zanzibar, and exotic but grown in Kenya, Malawi, and Mauritius. It is in the family *Curcubitaceae*, the same as the gourd, calabash, pumpkin, cucumber, and melon. It is not a tree but a liane or woody vine, capable of climbing as high as the tree canopy in a tropical forest, using the support of other trees. It has been commercially grown on plantations, typically planted in the drip line of existing trees. It flowers fifteen to eighteen months after planting, and the fruit ripens five to six months later. It produces up to thirty gourds in its third year, and continues to produce for twenty years. It is a drought-tolerant plant, frequently found growing up trees in lowland rainforest and riverine forests.

KEY FEATURES OF KWEME

>> Kweme is a liane that can only grow trellised or supported by forest trees.

>> Kweme oil is used locally in breast massage to encourage milk flow.

>> It is very high in extractable oil, containing as much as 61 percent oil.

>> Kweme seeds taste similar to almonds when roasted.

>> The benefits of kweme are derived from its concentration of essential fatty acids, polyunsaturated fatty acids, and iodine.

>> The seed oil is used for a number of domestic (household) and natural cosmetic formulas; like many of the other African oils discussed, kweme has a long shelf life.

>> Oils like kweme, high in EFAs (essential fatty acids), add luster to hair, and perhaps stimulate sluggish hair growth as well.

Theobroma Cacao (Food of the Gods)

The *Theobroma cacao* tree is as beautiful and intriguing as it is useful. One of the world's top economic botanical plants, *Theobroma cacao*'s pods yield cocoa butter, cocoa powder, and that delectable confection we all desire—chocolate. The *Theobroma cacao* tree grows in the tropical rainforests of Central America and Africa, particularly Côte d'Ivoire and Ghana, where it makes a significant impact on the local economy.

I recently saw a cacao; the tree is a remarkable sight. It has dark brown bark resembling the color of dark chocolate. Curiously, white flowers grow directly from the branches and trunk of the tree. Delicate, light-colored blossoms create a sharp visual contrast against the deeply colored, rough-looking bark. In fact, the cacao tree is one of the most unusual trees that I have seen. The scent the tree emits is quite subtle, not rich and chocolatey like you might expect.

THE MAKING OF COCOA BUTTER

Cocoa butter is created from the hydraulic pressings of cocoa nib or cocoa mass, from cocoa beans that are further refined through filtering or centrifuge. The scent of cocoa butter is removed using steam or a vacuum. Some herbalists, massage therapists, and aromatherapists prefer deodorized cocoa butter.

USING COCOA BUTTER

Cocoa butter is a useful ingredient for vegans (those who prefer to use no animal products, including beeswax), because it is a serviceable hardener, thickener, and counterbalance to stickier ingredients like shea butter. An additional contribution of cocoa butter is that no solvents are involved in its manufacture; it is a food grade, edible ingredient. The edible aspect is appealing to those who desire wholesome, nurturing ingredients in homemade potions, creams, and healing balms. Cocoa butter is widely available, ships well, is reasonably priced, and has a shelf life of two to five years.

Cocoa beans are 15 percent fat. The oil is very attractive as an ingredient in herbal cosmetics because it is cheap, readily available, and multipurpose. Cocoa butter has been traditionally used as a skin softener, emollient, pregnant and postpartum belly rub, and soothing substance for burns. It is useful as a superfatting agent in soap. To superfat cold-process soap, add half a teaspoon of melted cocoa butter per pound of soap. Of course, many soap bars double as shampoo and conditioning bars.*

Its high stearic composition allows cocoa butter to increase the hardness in handmade soaps and healing balms. In a pinch, I have substituted it for beeswax with good results. It can also be used as a base oil in soapmaking, where it is best combined with other oils, such as coconut oil, for a productive lather. The addition of tropical oils like coconut, palm, or almond oil helps create a looser healing balm or salve that melts faster. A hard soap, containing large concentrations of cocoa butter, lasts for a

---

*Superfatting is a process used in cold-process soapmaking, accomplished by adding liquid fat after the oils have been mixed together with lye. These oils tend to have more of a therapeutic effect because they have had limited contact with the lye.

long time in the bath. Cocoa butter–enriched soap will also hold intricate patterns in elaborate molds. Cocoa butter melts with body temperature, like shea butter.

BLACK COCOA BUTTER

One of my newest enthusiasms is black cocoa butter. Most of you are probably familiar with the eggshell-colored cocoa butter that has been widely available for quite a while, but this fixed oil is sold in several different forms. Most of the ordinary cocoa butter from Africa is processed before the seeds are allowed to germinate. With black cocoa butter, cacao pods are germinated first, which produces a deep, espresso-colored butter, smelling richly of roasted cocoa. You might find that as body butter it truly lives up to the botanical name of *Theobroma cacao*, "food of the gods." If you want to try something a little different in your skin-softening regimen, consider black cocoa butter, because it is softer and more malleable than the cream-colored type.

Black cocoa butter is very easily absorbed by the skin and is a nice addition to soaps, lip balms, and body butters. The dark color will temporarily stain light skin, but the oil is absorbed readily; once it is absorbed, no stain remains. It is useful as a hot oil treatment to condition hair. I purchase black cocoa butter from Terra Shea Organics, a supplier that buys its oils and butters directly from African cooperatives.

CHOCOLATE

Chocolate is derived from the same parts of the cacao tree, but it is processed, adding in other ingredients such as milk, which is also good for the hair and skin. This derivative of the cocoa pod contains flavonoids called catechins, which are very effective antioxidants. Dark chocolate, which has very little sugar, is preferred for health benefits, consuming as a treat, or applying externally in a spa treatment or hair care formula. Dark chocolate has 35 percent more of the brown paste of ground cocoa beans than other chocolate, so it is concentrated. The lactose in milk has been shown to help deter wrinkles, smoothing and refining skin texture. Lactose also acts as a good humectant, helping curly tops retain moisture in dry winter hair. The protein chocolate contains is boosted by the milk, making it good for unprocessed hair (without chemical relaxers or permanent colorants). I find chocolate with high cocoa content and low sugar a tasty treat that doesn't foil diet efforts.

WHAT'S SO GOOD ABOUT CHOCOLATE?

Nutrients in chocolate include:

≫ Protein
≫ Riboflavin
≫ Vitamin A
≫ Thiamine

The minerals:

≫ Potassium
≫ Calcium
≫ Iron
≫ Phosphorous
≫ Copper
≫ Magnesium

CHOCOLATE AND THE COMMUNITY

Many botanical-based beauty products containing cocoa butter and chocolate are available in spas, salons, and shops. As I mentioned, cacao is a huge economic boon to some countries; unfortunately, the way that this wealth is distributed is not always fair. It is best to buy chocolate products involved with fair-trade programs. Otherwise, you may be supporting child labor, or even the slavery industry that has cropped up in parts of Côte d'Ivoire around the chocolate industry. No organic chocolate products have been indicated in such unsavory schemes, so buy fair-trade or organic chocolate, cocoa butter, and cacao health and beauty products, avoiding the rest.

Savoring cacao's numerous health benefits is a nourishing treat for skin and hair, adding shine and vibrancy and improving the general health of both. By using chocolate and cocoa butter products on your hair and skin, you get to enjoy the delightful chocolaty aroma and reap the antioxidant, vitamin, and mineral benefits while skipping the fear of calories and guilt of overindulging.

> ### CHOCOLATE TRUMPS BOTH GREEN TEA AND RED WINE IN ANTIOXIDANTS
>
> Many of you are already familiar with the huge health benefits of green tea. You might not know, however, that cocoa has more flavonoids than green tea, which means that you are gaining a huge antioxidant boost from cacao-imbued products. In fact, chocolate may well have the highest amount of flavonoid available in a dietary ingredient. Using special analytical techniques to evaluate the total antioxidant content in each beverage, researchers found, on a per serving basis, antioxidant concentrations in cocoa almost two times stronger than red wine, two to three times stronger than green tea, and four to five times stronger than black tea.

Shea

You have undoubtedly heard a lot about shea, finding shea butter in your shampoos, conditioners, soaps, lotions, and creams. I find as an herbalist that it is always useful to also know where a particular ingredient, especially something as new to our marketplace as shea butter, comes from.

The shea tree is a member of the *Sapotaceae* family *Vitellaria parasoxa* C.F. Gaertin., formerly called *Butryrosperum paradoxum* (also used as a synonym). Shea trees are found exclusively in the African Sahel, a semiarid region south of the Sahara Desert. The shea tree is native to Benin, Burkina Faso, Cameroon, Chad, Côte d'Ivoire, Ghana, Guinea, Mali, Niger, Nigeria, Senegal, Sudan, Togo, and Uganda, where it is distributed in parklands, dry savannas, and forests. Shea trees grow between 150 to 200 years.

The nut of *Vitellaria pradoxa* is almost 50 percent fat. Shea butter is one of numerous nontimber forest products (NTFPs) that make significant contributions to rural African societies. Shea butter, known locally as *karite* in the Dioula language, is also called "women's gold" because it brings women significant income. Shea butter was traded as a commodity as early as the fourteenth century. Today, shea butter is the third-highest export product in Burkina Faso. It is one of the few economic commodities under women's control in Sahelian Africa. The trees have been tenderly cared for by women farmers and their children for hundreds of years, but, with the steady rise in the popularity of shea butter in international markets, some concerns have arisen.

Agroforestry and environmental organizations fear that overharvesting of the shea nut could contribute to land degradation, eventually leading to desertification. This is one of the reasons I also advocate using alternative butters like cocoa and mango butter as well.

While in the West we utilize shea almost exclusively as a cosmetic additive, in Africa it has diverse uses. For the Mossi people of Burkina Faso, shea butter is the sole source of vegetable fat. Groups in Burkina Faso and elsewhere use shea to make soap, healing balms, cosmetics, candles, lamp oil, and waterproofing putty for housing. Shea wood is used for creating tools, flooring, joinery, chairs, utensils, and mortars and pestles. The wood also creates a fierce heat and can be prepared as a substitute for kerosene, though the tree's destruction for fuel is discouraged because of its more prominent medicinal uses and and its economic contribution to African villages. The root and bark are used medicinally.

As I've said, many types of imported chocolates contain shea. Shea butter is exported to Japan and Europe to enhance pastry dough pliability and to enrich chocolate recipes. In Africa and around the world, shea butter is valued for its ability to soothe children's skin, soften rough skin, and protect against sunburn, chapping, irritation, ulcers, and rheumatism.

THE MAKING OF SHEA BUTTER

Creating shea butter from nuts is a monumental, labor-intensive task, involving huge amounts of water and wood, as it is made on an open-wood fire. West African Burkinabe women almost exclusively run the production of shea butter processing, along with the assistance of their children. Manufacture takes place during the rainy season, a time when harvesting duties are already intense for women. The preparation takes several days. Nuts are collected, boiled, sun dried, hand shelled, roasted, and then crushed with a mortar and pestle. Water is added and a paste is formed. Several women knead and beat the paste in a pot until a skim floats to the surface. The fat is cleansed repeatedly, yielding white foam. The foam is boiled for several hours. The top layer is skimmed once more and this yields the white shea butter we use.

I was so happy when shea became more widely available in the United States. I like using natural products that help support rural economies in Africa, and I appreciate the wide applications for this agroforestry product. Shea comes in many forms. A gold shea still smells of the woodfires on which it was processed. Pure shea is warm colored and has a good texture for kitchen cosmetics. White ultraprocessed shea is easy to use and is quickly absorbed into skin and hair.

Foraha: The Unique Restorative Oil for Healthy Hair and Skin

Foraha (*Calophyllum inophyllum* L.; family *Clusiaceae*) is also known as ballnut and Alexander laurel. Packed with essential fatty acids and crammed full of nutrients, it is garnering attention on the international hair and skin care scene as a miracle oil.

Foraha is a large evergreen tree native to East Africa, but it is distributed widely. It grows best in lowland forests or in coastal regions near forests. It is tolerant of various kinds of soil, including that of the coast, which is generally sandy, clay packed, or degraded. In addition to being native to East Africa, it is also native to tropical Southeast Asia, also growing in other parts of Asia and Oceania.

The fruit is called a ballnut. It is round and green, possessing a single large seed. As its fruit ripens, it becomes wrinkled, with color varying from yellow to earthy red.

The seeds produce a thick, dark green oil used medicinally or as a hair pomade. The pale kernel is sun dried for several months, becoming a sticky, dark, thick, and rich oil in the process before cracking. After it is cracked, it is allowed to dry some more.

FORAHA OIL

The seed kernel produces the precious oil, which is cold-pressed, yielding a greenish yellow oil with some similarity to olive oil, and a nutty smell. The oil is expensive, because the trees are very slow growing, and the full yield of the nuts of one tree is required to yield just eleven pounds of cold pressed oil.

There are many traditional uses for foraha oil in the annals of folk medicine where it grows. Primarily it is used for skincare. The tree and its medicines are thought to be regenerative.

≫ The leaves are soaked in water, and the resulting infusion is a blue brew that is applied to irritated eyes or consumed internally to treat heatstroke. The leaves are decocted, and the resulting tea is used to cleanse skin rashes and soothe hemorrhoids. The Manus people of Papua New Guinea infuse the leaves over an open fire. Once they are softened, they are applied to a number of skin disorders, including boils, cuts, sores, ulcers, and acne or other skin breakouts.

≫ Foraha sap, along with sulfur, formulates an ointment for boils, open sores, and wounds.

≫ Foraha oil is applied topically to scrapes, cuts, burns, insect bites and stings, acne and acne scars, psoriasis, diabetic sores, anal fissures, sunburn, dry or scaly skin, blisters, eczema, diaper rash, and herpes sores. Recognized as an analgesic, it is also used for sciatica, rheumatism, ulcers, joint pain, arthritis, bruises, oozing wounds, and chapped lips. Foraha oil is also used for several foot disorders, cracking skin, and foot odor.

≫ Centuries ago, Jamaicans used a type of foraha species to treat wounds and sores.

Foraha oil contains significant antimicrobial, antifungal, and antibacterial properties. It provides relief from the following:

≫ Abscesses

≫ Athlete's foot

≫ Bladder infections

≫ Boils

≫ Conjunctivitis

≫ Cracked nipples

≫ Diphtheria

≫ Bladder infections

≫ Eczema

≫ Infected burns

≫ Jock itch

≫ Madura foot, a malady that causes the bottom of the foot to swell and split

≫ Pneumonia

≫ Ringworm

≫ Septicemia

≫ Stings and bites

≫ Urinary tract infections

≫ Vaginitis

≫ Wrinkles (mature skin)

Foraha oil's chemical constituent qualities have been studied in numerous clinical cases. The fact that it can be used on burns makes it a welcome addition to African American and Latina hair care, or for others who chemically or heat-straighten their hair with flat irons or straightening combs. Foraha oil's ability to facilitate regeneration and act as an anti-inflammatory and antibiotic makes it a welcome addition to the curly hair care arsenal, particularly in protective and healing formulas for those who use heat or chemical formulas.

Not only is foraha oil recommended for skin disorders and scalp burns, its regenerative properties also make it the oil to reach for when trying to recover from hair loss or slowing evidence of the aging process. Many of us with kinky, curly, and wavy hair seek natural ingredients to help with hair growth or to stop breakage. In this area, foraha oil shows promise. In shampoo products, the saponification process releases calophyllic acid from the oil, which is highly restorative, so look for shampoos specifically containing foraha (also called tamanu oil). Foraha promotes new tissue formation, accelerating healing and inducing healthy skin growth.

You will notice that foraha goes by many names, so always look back to its botanical Latin name. Most commonly it is called foraha oil when it comes from Africa. It can be obtained from most quality online fixed-oil suppliers, soapmaking suppliers, and handmade cosmetic suppliers, and at your local health food stores. It is typically applied directly to skin neat (undiluted), though you may want to dilute it to save money. There have been some scientific reports of adverse effects from topical application (contact dermatitis), so do a twenty-four-hour test before using: apply a small bit to your wrist and see if there is a reaction the next day.

When building a trove of oils for nourishing skin or conditioning kinky, curly, or wavy hair, foraha should be included. As I mentioned, if you are using any type of chemical or electric straightener (relaxer, flat iron, straightening comb, or curling wand), reach for foraha oil to treat the burns that may occur. Foraha is renowned around the world for burn treatment. It is a wonderful aid for sistahs seeking relief from brand-new supertight cornrows, microbraid extensions, freshly twisted locs, or Nubian knots, which often produce a burning, itching, irritating sensation on the scalp.

Neem: Tree of Four Hundred Cures

Another miraculous tree is neem, an evergreen of the tropics and subtropics from the family *Meliaceae*. Neem has a distinguished history in India, documented in ancient treatises such as the *Atharva Veda*, the *Ghrhyasutra*, the *Sutragrantha*, and the *Purana*. In Sanskrit, it is known as *Nimba*, a derivative of the term *Nimbati Swastyamdadati* ("to give good health").[11] Neem has been naturalized over the past hundred years in coastal East and West Africa. Known as the Tree of Four Hundred Cures, neem is called *Mwarubaini* in the Kiswahili language.[12]

The leaves, seed kernel, and bark of neem trees are all useful. The tree has antibacterial, antifungal, antiviral, and infertility qualities. The neem kernels contain about 45 percent oil. The primary active ingredient is azadiractin, a bitter. Four hundred species of crop pests are affected by neem extracts, though it does not kill the insects but rather interferes with their biological functions and ability to reproduce. Compounds that lend these abilities include azadirachtin and nimbicidin.[13] Researchers from the International Centre of Insect Physiology and Ecology, Kenya (ICIPE), are using neem to tackle formidable natural pests in local farming. Scientist Ramesh Saxena, affectionately called the neem guru, leads a team at ICIPE to study the effects of natural pesticides used to control root-knot nematodes and fruit borers on tomatoes, and aphids and diamond black moths on cabbage. Neem is being tested as a deterrent to leaf miners, banana weevils, and ticks for postharvest grain protection as well.

Neem is an eco-friendly tree in more ways than pest control, as it contains compounds that inhibit the nitrification of the soil. In its natural setting, neem tree leaves quickly decompose, forming nourishing mulch.

Neem is used to treat ringworm and other fungal infections, particularly in medicinal manicures and pedicures. The emollient qualities of neem make it useful for treating skin and hair ailments. Apart from ailments, neem oil is also highly regarded for healthy maintenance hair and skin conditioner.

I insist on having neem on hand in my medicine cabinet. I use neem to quickly eradicate cold sores, to treat ringworm, burns, and hangnails, to soften cuticles, and on my feet, hair, and face. I give it orally to my children to treat viruses. Neem has what I consider a strongly nutty smell that many find unpleasant. Otherwise, it is your miracle cure: relatively inexpensive, becoming more widely available, and capable of addressing many vexing ills.

Akee: National Tree and Favorite Dish of Jamaica

I want to conclude this chapter with a very curious plant that could have simply been a poison. Poisons do have their uses, but instead it has become the national dish and national tree of Jamaica. The akee (*Blighia sapida*), called *akye* in Ghana, is a member of family *Sapindaceae*, the soapberry family. Native to tropical West Africa, akee grows in Cameroon, Gabon, São Tomé Principe, Benin, Burkina Faso, Côte D'Ivoire, Ghana, Guinea, Guinea-Bissau, Mali, Nigeria, Senegal, Sierra Leone, and Togo. The akee is related to lychee and longan. It is an evergreen tree that grows about thirty feet tall and has a short trunk.

This fruit tree was imported to Jamaica from West Africa, probably on a slave ship before 1776. Akee has become a major feature of various Caribbean cuisines. The word *akee* is thought to be of Twi language origin.

The flowers are unisexual and fragrant. They have five petals and greenish white blooms during warm months. The fruit is pear-shaped. When it ripens, it turns from green to a bright orange and finally to red, splitting to reveal three large, shiny black seeds.

The fact that West Africans, Jamaicans, and other Caribbean people have been able to make such great use of akee attests to their skill with assessing a plant's medicinal potential and usefulness, their careful preparation methods, and their ability to deploy effective detoxification methodology. Notably, the plant is used more in Jamaica than in its place of origin, West Africa; this indicates continuous, rigorous, ongoing development and maintenance of ethnomedical practice by black folk in the New World.

The aril of akee produce oils the essential fatty acids—linoleics, palmitics, and stearics. Only the fleshy aril around the seed is edible. The fruit and freakish-looking seeds are poisonous. The fruit must be picked after it ripens naturally, and it must not be overripe. Immature or overripe fruit are both poisonous. Even when ripe, it causes some to become violently ill, vomiting and becoming hyperglycemic; deaths have been reported, even by VIPs given akee in professional settings. Still, when prepared correctly, it is a wonderful dish.

In Jamaica, akee and salt fish is the national dish. In 2005 alone the akee industry was valued at four hundred million dollars. The arils are exported to the United States after undergoing rigorous testing to ensure they are safe for consumption.

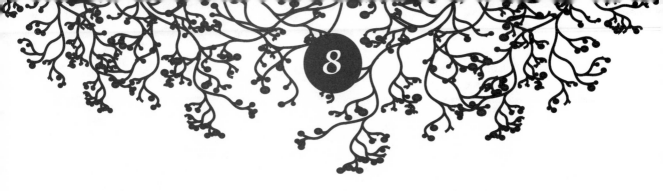

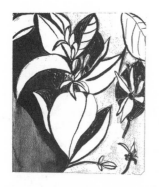

Fruit of Mother Nature's Labor

SOUL–NOURISHING BERRY AND FRUIT TREES

As I prepare for Kwanzaa, I set out gourds representative of *mazao* (crops) to contemplate a fruitful harvest. At the same time, our journey into tree medicine continues. My goal in this chapter is to broaden your perspective on fruit, showing ways that fruit trees and their leaves, stems, and oils are used in Africa, the Caribbean islands, and the Americas. This chapter presents new considerations for such familiar favorites as the peach and orange. We also explore fruits that may be exotic to some but are essential staples to others, from the time of enslavement and before, that deserve a second look.

Fruits from Africa and Africa's diaspora are some of earth's miraculous superfoods. Nuts, pods, and seeds from these trees produce luxurious oils and butters. Growing indigenous fruit trees helps many Africans preserve traditions and customs, solidifying collective identity and thereby restoring community. These trees support local economies and, because of their high yield for the amount of space used, conserve water, land, and labor.

IS IT A FRUIT OR A BERRY?

Fruits and berries are often confused. Berries are fleshy fruits with numerous seeds inside, like the banana, tomato, and pomegranate. What we commonly refer to as berries—the raspberry, blackberry, and strawberry—aren't actually berries at all; they are aggregate fruits, meaning they consist of a grouping of numerous smaller fruits.

One of my favorite decadent sweets is the date, a single-seed berry whose stone is made of hard, though edible, nutritious tissue. Dates are usually referred to as dried fruit, but they are actually single-seeded berries.

Juniper (*Juniperus communis*) berry is a spice used in Scandinavian cooking, an herb used by early African Americans and Native Americans, and one I use often making potpourri and incense. It isn't really a berry; rather, it is the female seed cone of the juniper tree. Juniper berries are also used to make gin.

My Banana God

A curious piece of folklore I carried to adulthood was always to cut banana with a spoon, not a knife. I never gave it a second thought until one morning I was having breakfast with some friends, who were very curious about why I was doing such a thing. They offered me a knife and I took it, a little embarrassed.

Why had my mother raised me not to take a knife to a banana? This is a piece of folklore of our people I've found elsewhere in my research, yet I can only speculate about its impetus. Earlier, when speaking of sacred groves of the Minianka, I mentioned that they are not allowed to enter the wood with anything that would be harmful to the trees, especially sharp cutting tools. Perhaps this is an Africanism retained and brought to the Americas by enslaved Africans. It wouldn't be the first.

Whatever the reason for not cutting them with a knife, I continue to look upon bananas with reverence. One of my favorite pastel paintings, "Banana God," was exhibited in West Africa in the Embassy at Cotonou. It was selected personally by the ambassador at the time, who said the pastel painting spoke to her and other people there because it focuses around the spirit in trees. "Banana God" makes an effort to illustrate the inner spirit of the banana. The banana is a cheap, readily available food with numerous uses. Whether in Kenya, elsewhere in Africa, Brazil, the Caribbean, or the Americas, black folk enjoy and rely on bananas. My sons bought a five-foot-tall banana tree for me as a Christmas present, to tend as an indoor plant. It is a gift that makes my heart soar—I truly relish its sight, particularly knowing all that it represents for African people.

One of the Baramago and Poko peoples' most potent spiritual medicines comes from the banana tree. *Mapingo* is a specialized tool, usually used only by a high-level regional diviner and only for the most serious problems. *Mapingo* uses the banana tree in divination. A device made of a horizontal banana tree trunk supports an array of short, small pieces of wood. They are arranged in groups of three and anointed with a medicinal mixture of palm kernel oil and other plant matter known to have specific metaphysical and medicinal qualities. The diviner petitions the sticks to answer the questions given. The answer is communicated by how the sticks fall.[1]

USES OF THE BANANA

The banana (*Musa paradisiacal var. sapientum*) is one of the most useful African staples. This multipurpose plant is used at home, as medicine, in utilitarian crafts, in ritual and ceremony, and even in cosmetics and trade. Portuguese or Christian missionaries probably introduced the sweet banana to Africa. It is cultivated in the forest regions and southern savanna area of West Africa. Nigeria and Côte d'Ivoire are major African banana exporters.[2]

Noble prize winner Wangari Maathai, founder of the Green Belt Movement (GBM), is a Kikuyu from Kenya, a people recently absorbed in intense tribal conflict over the Kenyan national elections. Before colonization, Kikuyu utilized the banana as a staple. The banana is an emblematic fruit, representing *harambee*, a Swahili philosophy that roughly translates to "let us all pull together."[3]

The fingerlike yellow delights are also fermented and used in other parts of East Africa to make alcoholic beverages. In Nigeria and Côte d'Ivoire, the banana brings economic returns as an export. Every part of the plant is useful.

- Banana leaves are used as animal fodder and to make umbrellas, roofing, tablecloths, and plates in Ghana. In parts of West Africa, poultices are made from large leaves to treat wounds. Banana leaves are used in ritual to bless babies and dispose of ritual and ceremonial items.

- The stem and peduncle (supporting stalk) of the banana yield useful fiber.[4]

- The inner peel contains antiseptic.

- Banana sap renders dye.

- Banana seeds are harvested and used to make decorative beads in Ghana.

- The fruit is consumed in many different ways: eaten raw, baked, fermented, and as a component in beverages.

In the New World, the banana is the beloved tree of Puerto Rico and other islands where people of African descent now live. Just as it is a staple in Kenya, in Puerto Rico the banana is so integral to the diet that it is referred to as poor man's bread. The roasted or fried banana is cooked, while the greens are served with other foods.

A wonderful gift of bananas, for that matter, is that they are very sustainable economical plants. According to Green Belt Movement (GBM), who champion its growth, one acre planted with banana trees can support fifty people, whereas an acre planted with wheat supports only two people. [5]

Eating bananas works wonders for the body in many ways:

> Bananas play a role in prevention of colon cancer.

> They improve colon function.

> They create good bacteria that ferments in your belly.

> They reduce high blood pressure.

> They reduce plaque formation in arteries (anticlotting).

> They help build bone density.

> They are a dense source of carbohydrates (energy).

> Banana acts as a natural diuretic, helping the body excrete water and sodium.

> Eating bananas can be useful for irregularity. [6]

> They can be a sweetener for hot cereal or baked goods, replacing or reducing cane sugar.

> Bananas are a useful addition to smoothies, adding body, fiber, good taste, and nutrition.

> They are a tasty addition to fruit salads with good texture, sweetness, and rich taste.

> Bananas make good emollient hair conditioners and face masques.

THE BRAT DIET

The banana is one of the milder, easier to assimilate, and digestible foods; as such, it is a part of the BRAT diet: Banana-Rice-Applesauce-Toast. This diet is typically recommended by pediatricians as a way to reintroduce foods to a child whose stomach has been upset by stomach flu, and those who suffer from diarrhea or vomiting. The BRAT foods are added one day at a time. Bananas come first, because they are a very safe, pleasant food for almost everyone. The banana is also one of the first solid foods introduced to babies.

BANANAS OF FIRE OR ICE

Here are two wonderful ways to enjoy the banana that fall at opposite ends of the elemental spectrum.

Frozen Banana

The frozen banana is the quintessential ingredient for smoothies and frozen drinks. It is also a wholesome, low-calorie replacement for ice cream, or can simply be a cooling snack. What could be easier? Peel the banana, cut it in half, and put the two halves in the freezer in a small freezer bag. Freeze until solid. Use as a delicious addition to smoothies or just eat them as is.

Grilled Banana

Place a firm (just ripe) banana on the grill with the skin intact. Turn with tongs until all sides are deep brown. Cut open and scoop out the roasted banana and place it on a dessert plate. Add a touch of cold whipped cream, with a sprinkle of cinnamon and a dash of nutmeg for contrasting temperatures, colors, and flavors. Eat immediately.

BANANA TREE

The banana tree is a lovely sight: sensually soothing, cooling, and inspirational wherever it grows. You will see banana trees in local conservatories in a city near you, or do as I did and request one as a gift to enjoy up close and personal. Banana trees live just fine indoors and are not fussy about water. They need about four hours of light per day. Of course, those of you who live in tropical regions know all about the banana's gift to the garden. Indoors or out, the banana takes us back through space and time to our ancestral roots.

Plantain

The plantain (*Musa paradisiaca*) is native to tropical Asia and was probably introduced to sub-Saharan Africa through Egypt. Plantains are not cultivated in East Africa, but they grow well there naturally. Beloved by Ghanaians, the plantain is cultivated in its forests and used as a staple food. In Ghana, there are twenty-one varieties in three main groups: *apantu*, *apem*, and an intermediary type between these two. Plantains are eaten in just about every imaginable way: boiled, eaten when unripe as *ampesi* or pounded into *fufu*, sometimes mixed with cassava. They are roasted and served with peanut butter, called groundnut, occasionally unripe but mostly ripened.

>> Fried ripe plantain is a favorite dish served with bean stew.

>> Unripe plantains are fried as chips, or dried and powdered as *kokonte*.

>> Ripe ones are pounded with corn dough and other ingredients and fried as *tatare* or *kakro* or used alone with porridge or as a sugar substitute.

>> Plantain stems yield fiber for fishing tackle.

>> Plaintains stems also make a sponge and towel used by elderly women.

>> Burned peelings of the fruit yield potash, used in local soapmaking.[7]

In Puerto Rico, firm green plantain is peeled, roasted, and fried and eaten in place of bread. At the popular Borinquen, or La Palma, restaurants in the Humboldt Park neighborhood of Chicago, this sandwich, called *jibarito*, is a guilty pleasure: garlic-seasoned, deep-fried green plantains with grilled steak or chicken, cheese, lettuce, tomato, and mayo. I enjoy it very much as a great occasional treat, replacing wheat flour, which is problematic for me and many others, with fruit. Take it a step further in the health direction by leaving off the mayo and cheese.

In savory dishes, plantain is roasted, fried, and combined with other foods. For the ultra-sweet tooth out there, wait until the plantain turns entirely black, advises my Trinidadian friend Gale, for an unsightly but unbelievable rich taste. Overripened plantains can be cut open, sautéed to a light golden color, and served over waffles with whipped cream, advises Michel, a friend from South America.

Flour is also made from plantains in Puerto Rico, by drying and grinding the flesh; this is used to make porridge or gruel. This kind of soul food helps most stomach disorders and is easily digested by babies.

For those unfamiliar, the plantain is similar to a banana, but starchier and less sweet, so they are often eaten cooked and served with savory dishes. The plantain is richer in vitamins and minerals than the banana, containing a daily value (DV) of vitamin C of 28 percent; 19 percent of the DV of B6; 10 percent of the foliate; 20 percent DV of potassium; and 20 percent DV of fiber.[8] I suggest delving right in. Buy one or two and experiment with them. I like them to be slightly soft to the touch through the skin, adding them at the last minute to savory soups, stews, or spicy sautéed curried dishes. Coconut milk accentuates this creaminess.

Fried plantain in place of potatoes for breakfast, or in a plantain sandwich, is how I learned to love them. As I write, I'm gazing at my three ripened plantains, with plans of sautéing them as a side companion to tonight's jerk chicken, with rice cooked in coconut milk, bay leaf, fresh ground nutmeg, cinnamon, and other delightful tree foods.

Clearly, the plantain is tasty and versatile as well as being packed with vitamins and minerals. A quick and easy Puerto Rican plantain recipe is to slice one and fry it in butter until brown, then sprinkle it with sugar, a pinch of cinnamon, and a pinch of ground nutmeg. For a healthier alternative, bake plantain whole until soft, then peel, slice, and serve as a sweet side dish.

Pineapple

Also called *pina*, pineapple (*Ananassa ananas*) is native to South America and is partially naturalized in tropical Africa and more extensively in West Africa. Wild varieties also grow in the African forest. Commercial crops are basically savanna trees, which grow particularly well in southern Ghana, where it is also important economically as an export.[9] In the Americas, Puerto Rico has long been famous for pineapple.

Some medicinal qualities of pineapple include the following:

> Sliced pineapple is placed in salt water before eating in Puerto Rico and West Indies.

≫ Pineapple juice is healing to catarrhal infections and is recommended for a sore throat.

≫ The stem and stump are rich in starch.

≫ Because it is high in the mineral manganese, pineapple has a very positive effect on regulating menstrual flow, especially when flow is too heavy. I advocate its use for smoother menstrual periods generally.

>> Manganese-rich pineapple strengthens bones; manganese is implicated as an aid to bone metabolism.

>> Ripe pineapples can be consumed juiced or eaten raw—pineapple juice is most easily absorbed by the body.

>> As an added bonus, the pineapple has a beautiful shape and color, which has come to symbolize the spirit of hospitality in many different cultures. This adds to its overall holistic health benefits.[10]

And here are a couple of additional easy and tasty ways of enjoying pineapple:

Grilled Pineapple

Peel the pineapple. Slice it width-wise in half-inch slices and place the slices directly on the grill. Sear each side for about four minutes. Eat as an accompaniment to seafood or fish or as a dessert.

Shish Kabob

The softening juices of the pineapple will tenderize meat or poultry as they grill, and the fruit also adds pleasing color. Peel, core, and cube a pineapple (make sure it is not overly ripe). Slide a cube of seasoned meat, a cube of pineapple, a slice of pepper (green, red, orange, or purple), and a slice of red onion onto a skewer; repeat until the skewer is full. Grill until the meat is cooked.

Pineapples are so easy to grow that in some countries the fruit itself is not sold because so many people grow the trees. To get your pineapple tree started, slice off the green part of a pineapple fruit. Let it dry for a few days, and then set it in a dish of water. Roots will form in a few days, at which time you can put the plant into some airy potting soil. This must be watered regularly until the roots take, and it needs to receive good sunlight for four to six hours per day (or use a grow light).

Mango

Mango (*Mangifera indica*) family *Anacardiaceae* (cashew family) is native to the East Indies and Burma and is now naturalized in tropical West Africa, having been introduced in the sixteenth century by the Portuguese.[11] In Ghana, it grows better along coastal savanna. Mango is one of the most productive tropical plants.

Very little goes to waste when considering mango. We know about the fruit, but many other parts of the mango tree are also useful. Mango contains protein, fat, carbohydrate, minerals, vitamins A, B, and C, amino acids, resins, natural sugars, and citric, tartaric, and malic acids. Of course, the yellow-orange flesh indicates it contains the phyto precursor to the antioxidant beta carotene.[12]

It can be eaten green, like a vegetable (nice shredded), or ripe as a fruit.

Mango tree bark yields gum, some tannin, and a yellow dye. The seeds, leaves, bark, and roots of the mango tree have varied medicinal uses.[13]

Mango is a healthful fruit that has been incorporated into African, American, and Caribbean cuisine. Peeling a mango proves difficult until one learns how. To peel, hold fruit with the narrow end pressed to a cutting board. Cut with a very sharp knife, going with the grain of the fruit. Remove the peeling as you go. Continue to turn the fruit until the skin is peeled all the way around. Cut quarter-inch pieces of the fruit off, one at a time, and place them into a bowl. At the center is the pit, which can be discarded.

The leaves of the mango tree contain saponins (natural sudsing agents useful for soap and natural detergents), glycerine, sterols, polyphenols, and benzoic acid and possess antibiotic properties.[14]

Mango's starchy kernels are edible when roasted, and the kernel makes a good butter, used as base for ointment.

MANGO OIL

The fixed oil of mango contains oleostearin, starch, and gallic acid.

Mango oil or butter releases salicylic acid, a pain reliever also contained in willow, used to make aspirin.

One of its most exciting alternate uses is as an oil or butter for health and beauty. Mango oil contains triglycerides with a high emollient quality, beneficial to skin and hair care. This oil has a slightly sweet scent. Creoles of the Greater Antilles drink a decoction of the flowers to treat heart disease and asthma.[15]

Sausage Tree

A truly fascinating specimen, the sausage tree (*Kigelia Africana* or *Kigelia pinnata*, family *Bignoniaceae*), or *Kigeli-Keia* as it is called in Mozambican Bantu, is a tropical species occurring in the eastern part of South Africa (such as Swaziland), Namibia, Mozambique, Zimbabwe, and northward as far as Tanzania.[16] It is called *Nufuten* in Ghana. It grows on riverbanks or close to rivers and large streams elsewhere in tropical Africa, from Eritrea to Chad and west to Senegal. As we have seen in a common thread throughout the book, many trees that grow near water are held in awe as magical healing vessels in Africa, the Caribbean, and the Americas, connecting ancestors, humans, deities, nature spirits, and community. Obviously, a tree that roots next to water is special.

The sausage tree is fairly erect, not branching a great deal, and where it does the tips of the branches remain very thick. In South Africa, it is one of the largest trees of the lowveld, though relatively short; its stems have a diameter of about fifty-nine inches, with a widespread crown.[17]

It is a deciduous fruit bearer that sheds its leaves in late autumn or winter, depending on moisture. The flowers are very curious looking, bright red and fleshy. In spring they open, remaining attached to the trees for as long as two months. They are set in whorls of three on a central rachis.

The sausage-shaped fruit of this tree grow up to twenty inches in length and four in diameter. The fruit is a dull greenish gray to pale brown, hard, and very heavy. The fruit hangs from a very long, sturdy stalk. Fruits fall in March and April, which can be a dangerous time of the year to be near the trees if you are unaware—ouch! They remain undamaged on the ground for many months after falling.

Anecdotal evidence suggests that the sausage tree's fruit has an ability to fight skin cancer and Kaposi sarcoma (an HIV-related skin ailment).[18] It also has antioxidant and anti-inflammatory properties.

South African people, Khoi and San as well as my ancestors the Bantu speakers, have a long history of using this tree to fight, treat, soothe, and attract or deter as the case may be. It is used to combat:

≫ Fungal infections

≫ Skin ailments such as eczema, psoriasis, and boils

≫ Serious skin ailments such as leprosy

≫ Ringworm, tapeworm

≫ Postpartum hemorrhaging

>> Diabetes

>> Pneumonia

>> Toothache

>> Piles (using boiled roots, stem, and bark)

>> Gonorrhea (using a decoction of bark)

>> Rheumatism[19]

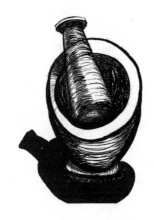

Some nonmedical uses:

>> Tsonga women use it as a cosmetic against the sun and for its antiaging properties.[20]

>> It is used as an aphrodisiac.

>> The fruit is used to ferment beer.

>> The leaves are used for livestock fodder.

>> Wild animals such as monkeys, baboons, and elephants eat it.

INTERNATIONAL USES OF THE SAUSAGE TREE

The seed oil, pulp, bark, roots, rind, and an extract of the fruit are all used medicinally. The sausage tree is used in the global marketplace for the following:

>> Research is being conducted to support the claim that sausage tree fruit extract is useful for skin cancer.

>> It is used in cosmetics to even the complexion.

>> It is added to "breast-firming" formulas.

>> It is used for wrinkle reduction.

>> It contains antioxidants good for stimulating hair growth and maintaining the natural condition of kinky, curly, and wavy hair.

>> It is an effective burn treatment.

>> It helps with pimples, razor burn, and other rashes.

>> Interest is developing in using the extract against skin infections.

Island Fruits

As you have seen, trees that grow in the tropical or savanna regions of Africa often grow equally well in the Caribbean, and many of those island fruits are widely available in the United States. Some remain unfamiliar, but you'd be wise to learn more about them.

GUAVA

A year or so ago, I tottered into Whole Foods Market with that feeling you get after tossing and turning all night due to stuffed nostrils, shallow breathing, and coughing. I was run down and depleted from a wicked cold. I ran into my friend Gale, who works there. I was reaching out to the shelves she lovingly stacks for something high in vitamin C, and she pointed me toward something unexpected, guava juice, saying it would give me the fix I needed. Shocked, but trusting her island wisdom and the fact that I've known her for over eighteen years, I tried it. Admittedly it did speed my recovery, tasting good at the same time. Later, I did some research to find out why she'd suggested it.

I came to find out that guava (*Psidium guajava*) is one of earth's most valuable fruits. It is much higher in vitamin C than citrus fruits like oranges or lemons, particularly if you eat its rind. It contains an appreciable amount of vitamin A, along with some iron and pectin, which is used to make jam and promotes digestion. The leaves and bark of the tree have a long history of medicinal uses. For example, an infusion of guava leaves or a decoction of its bark are used by traditional people to treat diarrhea, dysentery, and vertigo as well as regulating menstrual periods. Guava contains many wholesome natural chemicals.

In the Caribbean, it is known that guava has anti-inflammatory, astringent, and antihistamine properties and is useful for treating insect bites and hives. It is also known to fight bronchitis and kill viruses and is used in treating ulcers and boils.[21]

Guava juice is available as nectar or as 100 percent juice. I recommend the juice, chilled if desired, as a rejuvenating, wholesome morning drink as well as an elixir when you are feeling run down.

Virgin Bahama Mama

½ cup coconut milk

½ cup guava juice

Half a frozen banana

1 cup finely chopped pineapple

1 cup ice cubes

Place all the ingredients in a blender. Blend on medium-low for 15 seconds, medium-high for 15 seconds, and then high for 10 seconds. Drink immediately. Makes two eight-ounce servings.

BREADFRUIT: TREE OF SUSTENANCE, COMMUNITY, AND PERMACULTURE

The breadfruit (*Artocarpus altilis*) is an evergreen tree, growing roughly forty to seventy feet. Its canopy is spread. The trees begin to bear fruit at three to five years old and continue to produce for decades.

The fruit varies significantly in size, shape, and texture. Breadfruits are usually round, oval, or oblong, weighing about half a pound to thirteen pounds. The skin texture ranges from smooth to rough or spiny. Breadfruits are light green, sometimes with a tinge of yellow, yellowing more as they mature. The inner flesh is creamy white to pale yellow. The fruits mature and are ready for cooking and eating in fifteen to nineteen weeks. Breadfruit is a starch staple. The skin is soft, sweet, and creamy and can be eaten raw or cooked. The fruit can be seedless or have numerous seeds depending on the variety. The seeds are round or obovoid, with pale to dark-brown seed coats.

Breadfruit is a curious-looking tree from the Pacific. Today, it is an important cultivated tropical fruit around the world. In the late eighteenth century, several seedless varieties were introduced to Jamaica and St. Vincent during a time of famine, and a Tonga variety was introduced to Martinique. It is said that these fruit trees were imported as a high-yield, high-impact nutritious food to feed enslaved African workers. Purportedly, an original breadfruit tree from those times still stands, planted by Captain Bligh, in St. Vincent Botanic Garden. Polynesian varieties spread throughout the Caribbean, Central and South America, and Africa, including Madagascar. They also grow in south Florida and other locales. Its names in various languages attest to where it is appreciated most by Africans and people of African descent in the New World: Spanish *arbol de pan, fruta de pan, panapen, and pan*; in Benin *biefoutou, yovotevi*; Caribbean *cow, panbwa, pain bois, frutapan, and fruta de pan*; in Honduras *mazapan*; Tanzanian *shelisheli*.[22]

As one of the highest yielding fruit trees in the world, breadfruit is replenishing in many ways. A single tree can produce up to two hundred fruits per season. The fruit can be eaten cooked or raw in various stages of maturity. Breadfruit, particularly the seedless varieties, are grown as a subsistence crop in home gardens and farms. Used to replace starchy vegetables, pasta, or rice, the fruit can be baked, boiled, roasted, or steamed.[23] It is eaten as a dietary staple comparable to the plantain, sweet potato, cassava, white rice, and taro. Breadfruit is high in carbohydrates, yet low on the glycemic index. It is a good source of fiber, potassium, calcium, and magnesium, with small amounts of B complex and iron. Yellow-colored breadfruit flesh contains vitamin A. The seeds are edible and can be boiled, roasted, or ground into meal. They resemble chestnuts in flavor and texture.

Permaculture encourages the growth and maintenance of trees that are sustainable and that work well with their ecosystems without being destructive to the indigenous environment, and which provide the community useful functions such as shade, mulch, watershed, and fruit or nuts or other sustaining food sources for people and animals.

Breadfruit trees are very versatile, growing in a variety of conditions; if you don't live in the tropics, you can still see them in several of our country's conservatories (we have some here in Chicago). Not fussy about their conditions or treatment, breadfruit is a tree many amateur gardeners in tropical climates can grow.

The trees are important to traditional agroforestry, creating a protective canopy of overstory shade and understory mulch. The breadfruit tree provides watersheds, replacing slash-and-burn agriculture and field cropping with a healthy, productive tree that fits readily into the permaculturalists' vision.

Annona: Welcome to the "Family of Annual Harvests"

For those of us living in the United States, it isn't every day that we come across *annonaceae*, though, once you try them, you'll wish you did. Like the modern American family, this one is also in a state of flux; family *Annonaceae* is currently considered to consist of about 150 species. Still considered an exotic fruit here, these oddly shaped, fragrant, unique-tasting fruits are becoming more widely available, especially through fresh foods markets in Latino neighborhoods.

Annonas are small trees or shrubs. They have an erect habit, spreading moderately, with drab-colored grayish-brown bark that is rough or corrugated. There is a taproot, which is not as strong as other tropical fruits, and the rest of the root system has numerous thin lateral roots. The flowers are hermaphroditic and typically fragrant. Flowering begins when the tree is three to four years old. They are hand pollinated in cultivation, and in nature they are cultivated by wind or insects.[24]

CUSTARD APPLE

Known as *Condessa e coracilo-de-boi* in Portuguese and Bullock's Heart in English, custard apples (*Annona reticulata L.*) contain reticuline, which serves as an analgesic. Custard apple is a tasty treat used to make ice cream. Eaten on its own, it tastes like a mixture of banana and ice cream. The custard apple is considered an effective treatment for colds. It is also used to assist regularity in Jamaica.[25]

The leaf, stem, and bark of the custard apple tree contain acetogenins with cytotoxic potential, useful in cancer treatments.[26] The roots and stems have amino acids, and the fruits contain essential oils.

SOURSOP

The soursop tree (*Annona muricata*) grows to only about twenty feet tall. Its leaves are leathery, very dark, shiny, and green in color, and they exude a pungent odor when crushed. The tree yields yellow flowers. The soursop, also called *guanabana* or *mamon*, has an oblong, somewhat curved fruit, around thirteen inches long and weighing up to eight pounds. The fruit has numerous black seeds. The creamy, aromatic pulp is juiced and used to make ice cream. Soursop contains vitamin A and is rich in vitamins B and C. With its musky, acidic flavor, this native of tropical America is grown on small plantations or in private gardens. The fruit is high in linoleic acid and also contains unsaturated fats. The leaf and stem contain acetogenins that can be prepared as insecticides. The roots, stem, and leaves also contain acetogenins with antitumor activity.[27] In Cuba, a cocktail called *champola* is prepared using soursop. The soursop is a popular garden fruit in the Caribbean.

The soursop is used

>> For high blood pressure

>> As a sedative

>> As a central nervous system stimulant (to treat "nerves" in Jamaica)

>> For healing baths

>> As an antibiotic, antiviral, and antibacterial[28]

Soursop is also used in Suriname's traditional medicine:

>> A medicinal tea created from soursop leaves treats nervous tension and hypertension.

>> It is used as a treatment for flus and fevers.

>> The fresh leaves are used to alleviate insomnia.

>> The strong insecticidal action of soursop seed oil kills lice.[29]

Soursop Ice Cream

1 soursop fruit

¼ cup water

½ lime

½ teaspoon ground ginger powder

½ teaspoon vanilla extract

1 tablespoon sugar

1 can sweetened condensed milk

Peel the soursop and remove the seeds. Press the flesh through a fine sieve over a bowl. Add the water and place in blender. Add the rest of the ingredients and blend for 20 seconds. Pour this into a conventional ice cream freezer or ice cube tray. Freeze. Makes 1 quart.

The leaves are clearly medicinal, and soursop also contains phytochemicals in the seeds and stem, which fight several types of cancers. Remarkably, soursop appears to seek and destroy actively reproducing cancer cells while leaving the other cells undisturbed. Researchers are attempting to isolate the chemicals with the strongest anticancer and antiviral activity.

I first tasted soursop in Australia while on an exotic fruit tour along with my family. It is heavenly! Soursop eaten ripe without preparation tastes like ice cream, so imagine how tasty the recipe here will be. Beloved in the Caribbean, these rich ingredients come together to enhance the soursop's naturally creamy taste. With its hint of tartness from the lime and a dash of ginger providing spice, you'll find yourself returning for more.

SWEETSOP

The ripe fruit of sweetsop (*Annona squamosa*) is sweeter than soursop, with a good flavor and low acid.[30] Sweetsop contains borneol, and the fruit is used as an analgesic in Jamaica. Sweetsop contains acetogenins and fatty acids, and the seeds contain stearic, oleic, and linoleic acids and essential oils. The seeds are rich in acetogenins, and contain some saponin. Sweetsop also contains components to create pesticides and insect repellents.

The leaf is used to treat prolapsed anus, anal sores or swelling, and hemorrhoids. The root can be decocted and used as a purgative, a mild laxative, and a digestion aid.

WILD SOURSOP

As you can tell by its many local names—*Mchekwa* (Kishwahi), *nwitu, ntokw, mtokwe* (Kenya), *nchakwa* (Tanzania), *dauha, dyangara* (Bambara), *dugor, jorgut* (Wolof), *mulembe, mponjela* (Mali), *ntantanyerere, mtopa* (Zambia), *gishit'a* (Ethiopia)—wild soursop (*Annona senegalensis Pers.*) is a popular bush food in Africa.[31] It contains chemical constituents in its leaves that form insecticides. Wild soursop is rich in fatty acids, flavonoids, sterols, monterpenoids, and sesquiterpenoids. This bush fruit contains usable protein when served as a vegetable, and its seeds are also cytotoxic.

Wild soursop leaves, roots, and bark are used to fight cancer, convulsions, venereal disease, diarrhea, dysentery, fever, and impotency in males.[32]

Wild sourop leaves are infused to make a tea that treats eye disease and stomach and intestine disorders.[33] An alcoholic drink is made from wild soursop leaves that is used for its relaxant properties, as an antispasmodic, for soothing muscles, and for anti-ulcer actions.

ANNONA AS CANCER FIGHTERS

Obviously, annona is far more than an exotic fruit; its medicinal capacities need to be understood more in the international community. At the same time, key researchers who have pointed out family *annonaceae*'s tremendous health potential and benefits make it clear that, because of undesirable, potentially hazardous side effects when used as herbs, like most effective medicines these trees must be used with professional advice, not as a home remedy.[34] I am supplying this exciting information about their benefits because I am sure you will start seeing annona fruit pulp and herbal formulas, and I want you to understand what the fruits are, where they come from, and why they are so coveted.

Allspice and Bay

While visiting the islands, we'd be remiss not to consider the allspice tree, also called pimiento. Grown extensively in Jamaica, allspice comes from a small tropical tree that grows to about twenty-eight feet. Allspice (*Pimenta dioica*) is also called Jamaican pimiento, Spanish pimiento, pepper, or peppercorn.

The allspice is very important to Jamaican cuisine and as an exported spice, having grown there since around 1500 C.E.[35] We also receive allspice from Honduras. Allspice is a member of the fragrant-leafed *Myrataceae* family, to which myrtle, bay (as in bay rum and cologne), and cloves belong.

The allspice is a relatively small and shrubby evergreen tree, grown outdoors in the tropics and subtropics. It is tender and killed by frost, and can be grown in a container as a houseplant or in a greenhouse. This tropical evergreen tree has aromatic gray bark, leathery green leaves, and, most important to this conversation, dark purple berries. Allspice gets its name because it has a cinnamon, nutmeg, and clove aroma and taste. It is a dioecious tree, needing both male and female to produce fruit; when females mature, they yield berries if paired.[36] When dry, the fruits resemble brown, dark, smooth-skinned peppercorns that are larger than average, hence its nickname.

>> This spice is vital to Jamaican cuisine, North African and Middle Eastern foods, and American pudding, quick breads, sturdy cakes, stews, and barbecue sauce.

>> Allspice leaves and wood are used for smoking meats—the original *jerk*.

>> Allspice berries are ground and used in mole sauces, pickling, sausages, and curry.

>> Allspice essential oils are used in aromatherapy, as a tonic and tranquilizer, and for treating intestinal problems, depression, rheumatism, colds, and cramps.[37]

JERK AND ALLSPICE

Like its healing ways, Jamaican food hosts a historical confluence of Spanish, African, British, East Indian, Portuguese, Chinese, and Middle Eastern immigrants. These diverse ethnic groups come together to create Jamaican cuisine. West Indian Caribbean food depends heavily on herbs and spices such as the Jamaican scotch bonnet pepper. The signature ingredient, however, is the indigenous pimiento berry that we call allspice. Added to many dishes, savory or sweet, there wouldn't be any jerk as we know it without allspice. Jerk, as in Jerk Chicken, was made using the wood of the tree long ago. It was used to marinate wild boar as far back as the seventeenth century. Jerk is favored as much for its flavor as for its tenderizing effect and mouthwatering aroma on poultry, fish, and pork.

Allspice plantations are popular sensory destinations in Jamaica, and are great for romantic walks. Fresh allspice berries should be grated when green to release their full flavor. As an herb, allspice is used to treat chills, indigestion, and gas, and as a tonic.[38]

Pomegranate

Called *taroumant*, *armoun*, *tarmint*, and *aroumane* by Berbers, a group of indigenous North Africans; *Rumman* in modern Egyptian Arabic, and *inhmn* in ancient Egyptian, pomegranate (*Punica granatum* L.) is not a fruit but rather the berry from an African and Asian tree. Its original Latin name, *Arbor punica*, means "Carthaginian tree," named probably because the Romans first encountered large groves of pomegranate growing in North Africa's famed ancient city of Carthage. Rome waged war with Carthage, wars called the Punic Wars, a word also evident in its Latin etymology. Pomegranate's other Latin names are *Malum punicum* (Carthaginian apple) and *Malum granatum* (seedy fruit).

You have seen that many trees have numerous genus and species. This is not the case with pomegranate. Pomegranate only has one genus and two species. It is a small tree or shrub, growing between twenty and thirty feet. It is multiple branched, spiny, and extremely long lived, some reported as old as two hundred years. The leaves are either evergreen or deciduous and are leathery textured. Bold flowers appear on the branch tips, as many as five to a cluster. The seeds represent more than half the body weight of the fruit, and that is why I have place pomegranate in this particular section.[39]

Cultivated in Africa since ancient Carthage, which is in present-day Tunisia, pomegranate grows in tropical Africa and the East Indies. Pomegranate is commonly planted in Bermuda and is also grown in Honduras. This tree prefers a mild temperate and subtropical climate, but it adapts to regions with cool winters and hot summers; thus, it is grown as far north as Washington, D.C., but it doesn't flower there. It prefers semiarid conditions.[40] Because of its wide variety of uses as a tree, not just a fruit, this is a tree to consider adding to your garden if you live in the right temperature and climatic conditions.

Pomegranate fruits have such a singular appearance that they have sparked many a myth and legend. The rich red color lends the pomegranate uses in love magic. Vegans and others use its fruit juice as a substitute for sacrificial blood in offerings, rituals, ceremonies, and spells because of it resemblance to blood. Recently, the pomegranate has come into the media spotlight as a potential healer, but its history in holistic health is of a far greater vintage. It has been used medicinally since at least since New Kingdom Egypt (sixteenth century B.C.E.). Pomegranate continues to be widely used in North African medicine as a nourishing food.

Many parts of the pomegranate are useful. The bark of the root is antihelmintic, and the tree bark is a vermifuge. The root and bark can be decocted to release an astringent solution. This fruit tree makes a malleable wood, good for carving and other crafts. Walking sticks are often made from pomegranate wood.

The rind is especially astringent. Dried, pulverized pomegranate rind is used to treat ulcers of the digestive tract. It is antidiarrheic and hemostatic. Revered as a dentifrice, the rind is used to cleanse teeth, strengthen the gums, and fight plaque. The pomegranate rind and flowers yield important dyes used in textiles.

A contraceptive vaginal plug is made from pomegranate fruit. The fruit is also used to treat leukorrhea. The fruit is bechic, and used for pectoral troubles. It is a good preventative for airborne infections because of its cleansing (diuretic and astringent) actions. Ripe pomegranate is used to treat infections of the digestive tract.

An ink is created from steeped pomegranate leaves.

Parts of the entire tree are used in tanning and curing leather. Pomegranate bark has a 10 to 25 percent tannin content, the root bark is 28 percent tannin, the leaves 11 percent, and the fruit rind up to 26 percent. Pomegranate leaves, fruit, and peel are used for astringent properties and to stop diarrhea. The bark, stem, and root contain alkaloids used against tapeworm. The bark leaves and unripe fruit are astringent, halting diarrhea, dysentery, and hemorrhages. The leaves, roots, seeds, bark are hypotensive, antispasmodic, and anthelmintic.[41]

The flower buds are mildly astringent. Pulverized pomegranate flower buds are employed for bronchitis. The seeds show uterine-relaxing activity and estrogenic effects.[42]

A clinical update by Donald J. Brown, N.D., featured studies showing that the pomegranate fruit possesses a number of phytochemicals: polyphenols, luteolin, quercetin, kaempferol, and narigenin, found mostly in the fruit but also in the rind. Pomegranate seed oil is about 63 percent punicic acid, a rare trans 18-carbon fatty acid structurally related to conjugated linolenic acid. It contains the highest concentration of a specific phytoestrogen and is a potential cancer preventative. The pomegranate shows potential as a cardiovascular medicine and was found to reduce atherosclerotic lesions in some studies. The juice also possesses anti-atherosclerotic properties and decreases systolic blood pressure.[43]

Today, pomegranate is more widely available as a fresh fruit in local markets. It is also prepared as tea, juice, and ready-to-use pulp.

Plant some if you can. Read up on the pomegranate's unique place in mythology and folklore. Buy one. Peel it, section it, and enjoy its dense health benefits while knowing you are holding a revered fruit with an ancient African history right in the palm of your hand.

Home–Grown: Peaches and Oranges

Far from the exotic-looking pomegranate is the peach. We have plenty of peach orchards in the surrounding towns and counties of South Jersey, a few in Salem County, where I am from, and more in the counties that sandwich it, Cumberland County and Gloucester County, which are two of the Garden State's most prolific fruit and vegetable growers and processors.

Known as *Prunus persica* in botanical Latin, peaches grow in many different temperate and warm regions. The top peach producers in the United States are California, South Carolina, Georgia, and New Jersey. World-famous Georgia peaches owe their fame to folklore, heartwarming folk and blues songs, and recipes such as peach cobbler. From whichever region or source of inspiration, peaches are delightful seasonal fruits, brimming with vitamins, minerals, and fiber.

Peach trees are generally small; left to their own devices, they grow between twenty and twenty-five feet tall. In orchards, the shaped trees are kept much shorter through pruning. Peach flowers are delicate and pink.

The peach leaf has diuretic, expectorant, and sedative qualities. Peach tea (from the leaves) is used for chronic bronchitis and chest congestion. The leaves also have strong laxative action and are not recommended during pregnancy. The pounded leaves are made into a poultice and used to heal wounds. American folklore espouses the use of peach leaf for hair conditioning and hair growth, used as a water-based infusion. I have used a peach tea infusion with good results on dull hair that lacks body.

Peach Leaf Infusion

To prepare a peach leaf infusion, add 1 teaspoon of dried, crushed leaves to 1 cup of boiling water. Consume 2 to 3 cups per day.

Note: Peach tea has such a strong laxative action that is not recommended for use during pregnancy.

Using Peach Leaf as a Wound Healer

Add 1 teaspoon of crushed, dried leaves to 1 cup of water. Soak a square of gauze or a cotton square with the brewed leaves and tea. Use this as a poultice to aid a wound's healing process.[44]

For one practical idea, take a dried, cleaned peach pit and keep it on your person or in a mojo bag with other love draw herbs, stones, and ephemera as a love charm.

Peaches contain a lot of boron, which boosts steroids in the blood. The boron in peaches increases estradiol 17B, the most active form of estrogen, making the fruit useful to consume during menopause or after a hysterectomy. Peaches, because of the boron they contain, are believed to decrease occurrences of osteoporosis and increase testosterone.[45] I can attest to peaches' efficacy with menstrual cramps and PMS. They are also good for perimenopausal and menopausal symptoms.

We hear the most about peaches outside the kitchen when they're used as a cosmetic aid. Peach kernels are pressed, yielding precious sun-kissed and straw-colored oil that is not greasy. Peach kernel oil contains minerals including boron, as previously discussed.

I have always had very sensitive skin, and, unfortunately, I didn't really start to have acne until my childbearing years. Peach kernel oil is a delicate oil, suitable for those with skin like mine that is hypersensitive to artificial ingredients and fragrances. Peach kernel oil's regenerative and tonic abilities are attributed to its antioxidants, vitamins A and E, and minerals. It is also high in essential polyunsaturated fatty acids. It is used as a carrier oil in aromatherapy, and as an emollient hair or skin treatment. Recommended for its ability to battle dehydration, peach kernel oil is also respected for smoothing wrinkles and lending suppleness to all skin types. It is also recommended for inflamed skin, overexposure to sun and wind, and for serious conditions such as eczema and psoriasis.

PEACH TINCTURE

Buy prepared peach leaf tincture, and take 2 to 15 drops in water 30 minutes before meals.

The use of peach kernel oil in hair care formulations is similar to its use in skin care. It acts as an emollient, and it is so light that it is easy to wash out and won't weigh down thin hair. By coating the hair shaft, peach kernel oil helps hair retains both natural color and chemically applied color, making treatments last longer. For the same reason, peach kernel oil protects hair from environmental conditions such as sun, wind, rain, and pollution. Coating the hair shaft with light oil also deters frizz and helps define curl patterns. Nutrient-rich peach kernel oil or a peach leaf infusion conditions hair, aiding growth by preventing breakage and tangles.

Peach kernel oil can be used neat (applied to the scalp, hair, or skin straight from the bottle), but that approach may prove expensive. Most formulators, aromatherapists, and soapmakers, including this one, dilute it.

Remarkably, it is equally effective in dilutions of 10 to 50 percent in carrier oils such as grapeseed, sweet almond, or jojoba oil as when it is used alone.

To use it as scented carrier oil for massaging the head, scalp, or body, stir ten to twelve drops of pure essential oil into six to seven teaspoons of peach kernel oil. Recommended essential oils for kinky, curly, or wavy hair include sage, rosemary, lemongrass, lavender, Roman chamomile, sandalwood, palmarosa, patchouli, ylang/ylang, and neroli. You can pick a few and mix them, if desired.

Do-it-yourselfers will enjoy the superior emollient qualities of peach kernel oil when added to handmade creams, lotions, massage oils, and lip balms. Luckily, rather than slaving over a hot stove, these formulas are now pre-prepared and sold as ready-to-use bases by certain companies.

Of course, for best results, peach kernel oil needs to be kept out of the sun and stored in a cool, dry place, where it lasts for an incredible two to three years. The oil should also be derived from cold-pressed kernels, as overrefining reduces its beneficial antioxidants.

Warning: Anyone with nut allergies in the home should avoid peach kernel oil and products containing it.

Another interesting application for peach kernel oil came to light through a collaborative study between U.S. government scientists at the Agricultural Research Service and South African and Israel/Palestinian colleagues. It was found that the natural oil in peaches that lends their scent also kills fungi and other pests in soil. It is being investigated as a safer pesticide for animals, people, insects, and the environment.[46]

Many makers of handmade soap and cosmetic formulators, both commercial and small-scale entrepreneurs (whom you will find listed in a collective such as the Handmade Soapmaker's Guild), use nature identical oil (NIO) or synthetic peach scent (fragrance oils) for scenting candles, soaps, creams, lotions, conditioners, shampoos, and pomades. In aromatherapy, peach scent lends thoughts of peacefulness, gaiety, and romance, hence its use as an aphrodisiac.

ORANGE AND COMMUNITY

We survive and navigate the urban forest through community. Whereas traditional African women keep track of village goings-on while grinding plants into flour at the mortar and pestle, for us it is mainly done on playgrounds and at coffeehouses. Still, what we have in common is that these conversations with our sisters across the Atlantic are largely centered on family—our children and relatives, and their hopes and dreams—and on how things are and how we want them to be. Whether rural village, suburb, or city, we strive to build collective consciousness through story, and this is healing.

On the playground and in the coffeehouse, I have shared and have heard my sisters share their pasts, presents, and desired futures. We talk through our pregnancies, illnesses, and graduations, deaths in the family, a lost job or a new job prospect, a trauma, or just what's cooking for dinner. Sisters in Oak Park talk deep, and this is one of the healthy things about our tight-knit community. One such interchange took place with my friend Jan. New to our area, Jan has chocolate-brown skin, a slight southern drawl, close-cropped red hair, and a very fit body—she walks just about everywhere. When I told her about writing *A Healing Grove*, she got very excited. As our children played on the playground, she recounted her childhood story. She made me think of trees in a totally different way.

When Jan was growing up in Florida, her family knew that, no matter what, they'd never go hungry. Her grandmother and mother, two resourceful women, fed all the neighborhood children who would stop by, hungry from running around and playing, from the trees. The trees she grew up with were mango, grapefruit, and orange.

Florida oranges are world famous. In fact, while in these pages we've seen that many trees grow well in diverse parts of the diaspora, these delightful fruits grow best in that state. After our conversation, I wondered if oranges ever grow wild outside a place like Florida.

The orange tree is unknown in its wild state. It is believed to have been brought to the Mediterranean from southern China or northeastern India, probably by Portuguese explorers. Spaniards introduced it to South America and Mexico. The French brought it to the United States by way of Louisiana, and from New Orleans it was distributed to Florida around 1870. The rest is history; the orange is one of the most popular trees in the world, and the most commonly grown. It grows in the Mediterranean, in South America, the Caribbean, Egypt, Brazil, Jamaica, and in Louisiana, Mississippi, Alabama, and Georgia in the United States. Subtropical rather than tropical, it grows in a temperature range of thirty to fifty degrees Fahrenheit. Florida has the best conditions for growing this fruit, and remains the world's top producer.[47]

Outdoor orange trees grow on average to about twenty-five feet, but can grow up to fifty.[48] They have a rounded crown and slender branches, and the twigs are twisted and tangled when young. The leaves are aromatic and evergreen.

The fruit comes in a range of shapes, from globose, subglobose, oblate, or somewhat oval, and is usually 2½ to 3¾ inches wide. The skin is dotted with minute glands containing essential oils. The outer rind is orange or yellow when ripe, the inner rind, called pith, is white, spongy, and bland, and the pulp is yellow or orange. The fruit is tightly packed with membranous juice sacs, of ten to fourteen wedge-shaped sections that are easily separated. [49]

Those with small gardens in temperate zones and urban gardeners will appreciate the opportunity to grow fruit in their living rooms. The smell of most fruit trees is intoxicating, delicate, and light. Their cheerful sight, as they bear fruit, is uplifting. Citrus has the spiritual quality of cleansing foul vibrations and adding to the general holistic health of the environment. Recommended types for beginners are:

» **Sour Orange** Var. *Calamondin* or *Rangpur Lime*: The tree has wide, pretty leaves and produces bright orange fruit, like tangerines with a sour taste.

» **Lemon** (one of the easier types) Var. Meyer Improved dwarf, "Lisbon" or "Ponderosa" dwarf: Disease resistant, and requiring less heat than other citrus to produce fruit, Meyers' variety (*Citrus meyeri*) is very well suited for growing in containers. It bears fruit heavily with minimal effort. These juicy lemons are deep yellow, flavorful, and slightly sweet.

» **Kumquat**: With sandalwood-scented flowers, kumquat makes a good marmalade. Var. *Fortunella Margarita* and *F. japonica* as well as *F. crassifolia*; of the varieties available, *F. crassifolia* are round and sweet—good eating fruits.

» **Mandarin orange** (*Citrus reticulate*): Produces a mandarin-like fruit. Mandarin orange trees require less heat to ripen than a true orange, and can bear three to four crops per year indoors.

Many different types of hydrosols and essential oils are created from specific parts of various orange trees. Essential oils and hydrosols extend the use of tree medicines, lending environmental, healing, blessing, remembrance, cosmetic, hair care, and perfumery use. All this diversity comes from the ordinary edible orange.

Eating fresh oranges is good for us, better in fact than drinking the juice, because the whole fruit has more intact fiber and phytonutrients. An orange also has fewer calories than a serving of juice. Oranges make a tasty addition to fruit salads, such as ambrosia and the popular Harvest Salad, which contains dried cranberries, oranges, bleu cheese, and walnuts or sunflower seeds, with balsamic dressing. The zest and fruit make a nice addition to cranberry-orange walnut bread as well. My grandfather took advantage of the essential oils in the rind by chewing the skin. He found it to be a good dentifrice, refreshing the breath.

The sweet orange has been used as a substitute for soap and for washing clothes.[50] Orange wine was made in the old days by Floridians. Slices and peels were and remain a confection.

Rubbed on the face for acne, orange juice is beloved as a health cure-all due to its bioflavonoids, inositol, rutin, and vitamin C. Orange juice is also used to treat catarrh.

Orange nectar is more abundant than any other fruit source in the United States. Honeybees make light-colored honey from oranges, and 25 percent of all honey in the United States comes from the orange.

Roasted orange pulp can be used as a poultice for skin diseases.[51] The pulp in the juice is a good source of fiber.

The orange tree is made of a handsome wood that is close-grained, whitish to pale yellow, and hard. Walking sticks are made from orange wood in the United States, and in Cuba baseball bats are made from the orange tree. Orange wood is used also by manicurists as cuticle sticks.

Orange oil is derived from orange seeds, used for cooking, soapmaking, and to create plastics. Today, housecleaning formulas such as wood polish and botanical dish and laundry soaps continue to feature orange essential oils because of their pleasant, uplifting scent, with some broad-spectrum cleaning applications. A very positive attribute of sweet orange essential oil is that it is good for the spiritual and ecological environment. Whereas some essential oil is very expensive, sweet orange essential oil is affordable for students and those with limited incomes. I keep a large bottle of sweet orange oil on hand because of its practical applications within the home.

The soft nature of neroli lends itself to handmade soap. As a first step into soapmaking, purchase readymade blocks of unscented soap, called melt and pour (MP) soap. These soap blocks, sold by the pound, are prepared using a variety of ingredients including palm and coconut oils, aloe vera, olive oil, shea butter, hemp, honey, or even oatmeal. Follow the manufacturer's directions. If you enjoy color, add orange soap chips or even an orange crayon in the last stages of melting the soap. Add the recommended amount of essential oil (neroli). You can enhance the orange scent further by adding three tablespoons of orange blossom water during the melting stage.

As a neat alternative, pour melted and scented soap over loofah sponges cut into one-inch slices and placed in a metal or Pyrex baking dish. The loofah sponge is a vegetable skeleton with unique exfoliating qualities. Most recipes create at least a dozen bars of soap—consider giving some away. Orange blossom soap makes a great gift and only takes a few hours to complete. Wrap the soap in clear wrapping paper and seal with a festive ribbon.

PETITGRAIN

As you have seen with many of the fruits presented in this chapter, it is not only the fruit but also the leaves, stems, bark, and sometimes roots that are used medicinally. This holds true with orange as well. Petigrain is a uniquely scented essential oil with a deeper, spicier, and mintier scent than you would expect from the citrus family. It is made from steam-distilled or pressed leaves, twigs, and the unripe fruit of *Citrus aurantium*, used in skin and hair products, natural home cleansing, potpourri, and other creative ways in the homes, mostly of Westerners.

The key qualities of petitgrain include:

> ≫ Uplifting

> ≫ Has a supportive psychological and spiritual effect

> ≫ Relaxant for insomnia and tension

> ≫ Regenerating for convalescing and weariness

ORANGE: HISTORIC AND FOLKLORIC OVERVIEW

We are most familiar with oranges as the juicy fruit consumed during our daily waking rituals. Orange juice, not coffee, is one of the most invigorating, replenishing breakfast drinks, bringing energy to start the day.

A symbol of Sun Ra, the orange plant is one of nature's most vitalizing gifts, rich in possibilities for healing. As you have seen, many parts of the orange tree are used for holistic healing and complimentary therapies, and one of the most intoxicating is the blossoms, as you'll see in a bit.

Early enslaved African people made great use of sour orange, consuming it raw and smoking it (cooked in wood ashes).

Early African Americans also used it for dressing old wounds, veterinarian medicine, stopping vermin from entering wounds, and as a vermifuge.

Sour orange wood is attractive and used in small woodworking, such as walking sticks, by southern African American carvers.

Oranges in Suriname are of three different types: sour, bitter, and sweet. Originally from Spain and Portugal, they grow readily in warm to tropical regions of the Americas and Africa. Sour orange is used to treat sores and running ulcers in Surinamese folk medicine. Though it may sound exotic and relatively strange to contemporary ears, sour orange is the source of coveted neroli oil.

ORIGINS OF NEROLI

Neroli is one of the world's most expensive oils. It originated in the Far East and is believed to have been introduced to the Mediterranean by Arab traders. It has intimate ties to both Eastern and Western culture, especially royalty, making its true name origin hard to decipher. It is said that the word *neroli* is derived from *naranj*, which means orange in Arabic, or from the Sanskrit word *nagaran*. Thanks to the

Moors, neroli oil made its way further north and west. Production of this highly prized essential oil began in twelfth-century Spain.

There are differences between neroli and orange blossom water:

≫ The delicate blossoms, rather than the fruits, are used to create the pale yellow neroli from *Citrus aurantium*, *C. brigaradia*, and *C. vulgaris*.

≫ Orange blossom water is a by-product of oil production, created from *Citrus bigaradia* or *C. aurantium*.

≫ Neroli is steam distilled, whereas volatile solvents are used to extract orange blossom oil. Neroli is strong and long lasting.

≫ Neroli essential oil's origins are in the Far East, but it is now cultivated primarily in Italy, Tunisia, Morocco, and Egypt from steam-distilled blossoms of the bitter orange tree.

Here are two antiwrinkle astringents for the face made with orange products:

Neroli Astringent #1

3 ounces orange flower hydrosol

1 ounce witch hazel

1 tablespoon apple cider vinegar

Mix ingredients in a nonreactive bowl. Pour through a small funnel into a 6-ounce bottle. Dab on skin with a cotton square, thoroughly cleansing.

Neroli Astringent #2

This is another easy-to-make astringent, made by adding about 8 to 10 drops neroli to 16 ounces witch hazel in a nonreactive bowl and funneling into a clean, dry bottle. This is immediately ready to use; just shake very gently before application. Apply to the scalp (in the parts) or all over the face, working upward with cotton squares, to cleanse, soothe, and calm the nerves.

Antiwrinkle Mature Skin Oil

To a quarter-cup sweet almond oil, add 12 drops of neroli essential oil. Swirl to blend. Pour through a funnel into a 6-ounce sterilized dry bottle with a screw cap. Dab on the face with a cotton ball at night before bedtime.

Alluring Aphrodisiac Oil

1 cup sweet almond oil

15 drops neroli

10 drops sandalwood essential oil

Add ingredients to a nonreactive bowl in the order given. Swirl gently to mix. Using a funnel, pour into a clean, dry, 6-ounce bottle with a flip top. Use as a massage or intimate oil.

Other uses for neroli include:

» Neroli is a skin texturizer; it improves varicose veins, skin elasticity, and the development of new skin cells. It softens skin, lessens the appearance of wrinkles and scars, may regulate oiliness, minimizes enlarged pores, and clears blemishes.

» Neroli's antioxidant properties boost and revitalize dull-looking hair.

» It is helpful in treating many types of dermatitis and scalp irritation.

» It calms rashes.

» In matters of the heart, neroli is a purportedly effective aphrodisiac, alleviating sexual tension, and is also a cardiac tonic.

PRECIOUS OIL

Neroli oil is the extracted essential oil of fragrant blossoms from the sour orange tree. Like rose oil, neroli essential oil's expense is driven by the enormous amount of blossoms necessary to produce it. In fact, one ton of orange blossoms is required to produce one quart of neroli oil. However, before the orange blossoms are distilled to produce essential oil, all traces of debris, including green leaves and twigs, must be removed by hand. I keep a small bottle at the ready to use, add to facial creams, and use as a calming agent. When I plan to add neroli to potpourris or soaps, I generally purchase a sample, which is about one-sixteenth of an ounce, because it is very expensive.

Some uses for orange blossom water include:

≫ Orange blossom water can be poured into a suitable glass (crystal) or ceramic dish and placed on an altar for remembrance.

≫ Orange water is used for spiritual blessings.

≫ In Africa, the water is used in a refreshing, easy-to-make soft drink.

≫ It elevates the mood when used as an air freshener.

≫ Orange blossom water makes a great moisturizer and soother for the skin and hair.

EAST MEETS WEST: AYURVEDA AND AROMATHERAPY

In South Africa and Jamaica, Asian medicine is well integrated into practice. Best for the rest of us to get on board, and neroli offers a passport. In India's yogic tradition, neroli is associated with the second chakra, the sacral spinal area. Yogis and other practitioners of ayurveda admire neroli for its trance- and sleep-inducing qualities. It is rubbed on the abdomen or sacral area. In Chinese medicine, neroli is used to mobilize chi. Westerners used it aromatherapeutically to alleviate depression and to soothe anxiety, hysteria, and nervous conditions. Neroli addresses a variety of ills, including insomnia, anxiety, depression, diarrhea, and a broad range of menopausal issues.

BERGAMOT

Bergamot is made from bitter orange, *C. aurantium, var. begamia.* You are familiar with bergamot if you drink Earl Grey tea. It was also very popular as the scent in Afro Sheen and other hair pomades or pressing oils, sold simply as Bergamot. The greenish-yellow oil is extracted from the peel of the unripe fruit, crushed leaf, and twigs, releasing a fruity yet floral scent. Bergamot essential oil is recommended to treat grief, depression, anxiety, skin infections, and pimples, and for colds and influenza, and it has antiseptic qualities.[52]

To conclude this chapter, I want to share a wonderful ritual that was posted by a friend I made in the virtual world through the Yahoo group I moderate, the International Clan of the Eclectics. This soul-rejuvenating ritual shares ways to engage tree energy.

I have made a wonderful cleansing ritual with water and the nature spirits and plants from my yard. I carry a large pot as I walk around the yard at Moonhaven, which is a cross between a park and a jungle full of amazing plants, trees, and energies. As I move through the yard, I allow the elementals and devas to guide me to special trees in bloom. I gather pieces, leaves, flowers, buds, etc., from them into my pot, adding pieces of pine bark, needles, and cones. I always make it a point to add bark, leaves, and acorns from the most sacred Grandmother Tree, which is a 500+-year-old live oak that was struck and split down the middle by lightning some 300 years ago and still stands like an amazing Goddess sculpture alive and thriving. I believe that her energy infuses the entire magical space here at Moonhaven! Also in the mix are leaves and blossoms from my orange, tangerine, and lemon trees. Next I cook the harvest for about 20 minutes letting the aroma fill my house. Then I let it cool a bit and strain it into another pot and maybe add a bit more water to make it a pleasing temperature. This is usually done best with another so if you both want to receive these sacred waters, then be sure that you have enough mixture for 2 full large pots (like the kind you would boil up pasta in). Because I live in the country, this next part is easy but you could also stand in your tub or shower. Get naked and have your partner (or yourself) pour the magical tree water mix over your head. I also like the feeling of having some of it literally thrown at me to shake loose any remaining negative energy forms that might still be hanging on to my body. Blot dry with a clean fluffy towel and light a white candle and bask in your renewed energy. I do believe that a spring bath is just what this Witch Doctor needs!

—Flash Silvermoon, Dianic priestess and author of *The Wise Woman's Tarot*

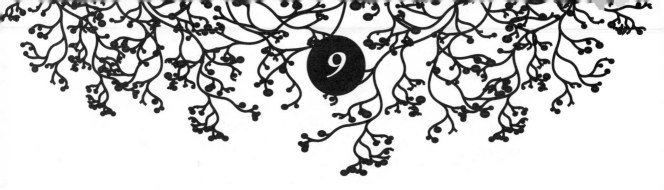

Bark, Gum, Sap, Resins, and Moss Medicine

Every healer is presented with a portal at some time in life; my portal had two entrances. I've written quite a bit about the influence of my environment—the woods, the lake, the rural environment of the New Jersey Pine Barrens as my spiritual and creative incubator. The second portal on my path was my parents.

Growing up, the two of them scared the living daylights out of me. My mother suffered with serious asthma and acute hay fever. There were too many occasions when she stopped being able to take in our most vital element: air. As a child, it was terrifying to see my mother struggle for her life, again and again, as I stood wide eyed, small, and powerless. My father had a lifelong heart ailment, brought on by a bout of childhood rheumatic fever. While I was growing up, he had several major heart events, including a heart attack when I was home alone with him; I was eleven or twelve. It was traumatic for us both. I somehow dropped his nitrobids behind a very large, immovable bureau—thankfully, he survived. If left to their own devices, children don't like to think about death or mortality. Like the dresser behind which the heart medicine fell, for my brothers, sister, and me, there was no way around facing potentially lethal illness.

The combination of my parents' illnesses and my bucolic outdoor environment put me on the path of healing. I always saw healing as holistic. For me, this means combining arts, as well as mental and spiritual energy, with herbalism, and applying it to all sorts of ills. I knew healing outside a hospital or doctor's office was possible because of stories I heard of my grandmother, who had passed on before I was born. She seems to have been able to calm, cure, and offer hope to many.

Grandma Edwina was a spiritualist minister: an old-style African American healer. My grandmother Lucille, who was alive during my youth, was gifted with divination: especially dreams, card readings, and tasseology. Anyone familiar with my writing knows that my uncle was an Afro-Cuban-style drummer and drum maker, a practicing Santeria *babalawo* under Elebga.

Decent holistic healer pedigree or not, just invoking the memory of my parents' struggle with their various illnesses, and remembering the dreaded fifteen- to twenty-five-mile drive to the hospital, depending on whether or not we went out of state, still makes my breath shallow and my heart beat too fast. As a yogini, I am always aware of breath, knowing that balanced breathing (taking in as much breath as you release), nice and even, calms the body, keeping it nourished and well. I don't like to "go there," as they say, into this frightening childhood memory. I'm going to take a deep breath right now and trudge along with this story, one I share only because this chapter connects to those times. You see, it is largely the outside parts of the tree that help people like my parents. Complementary alternative medicine (CAM), uses barks, saps, and resins to treat asthma, COPD, heart disease, and cardiovascular disorders.

My first trip into the portal revealed that white oak and wild cherry barks were good for my parents. Pine has also been used to help with coughing disorders. It is also an allergen, yet my mother loved it, and who is to argue when someone isn't well? These are the sorts of conundrums herbalists face all the time. Willow bark and leaf, the plant origin of aspirin, has some very useful applications to specific types of cardiovascular disease and is also useful for mitigating pain. These are great American trees, in ample supply in South Jersey, and they were my first teachers once I stepped through the healer's portal.

When dealing with a couple, often one person is open to integrative healing and the other one is not. During my youth, my mother was more trusting of medicine from the pharmacy and spirit dispensed at church pews. I think her indifference toward plant medicines might be because it was plants—new-mown hay, ragweed, pollen—that set off her allergies and her coughing, making her miserable and eventually kicking up her asthma. I do recall Ma had a special brand of hatred for goldenrod and its pollen. My father, on the other hand, was very much the outdoorsman, uncomfortable in church at that time and very open to herbal healing throughout his life. One certainly doesn't have to choose between religion and herbs, but that is not my point. As we've seen with the examples of Jamaican healers, some of their paths integrate Christian prayer, energy work, and herbalism quite readily, and this also occurs elsewhere in the diaspora.

In South Jersey, I looked to our notable American medicine trees for their healing potential. Elsewhere in the diaspora, my story would have been different—your Tree Medicine Kit is greatly influenced by the patch of earth on which you stand. Baobab would be one of the best trees to illustrate a multiuse tree elsewhere. Every part of that tree is useful with purposes in the African village. You could call it a coffeehouse, meeting hall, funerary lodge, birthing suite, shaman's office, water cooler,

> *Your Tree Medicine Kit is greatly influenced by the patch of earth on which you stand.*

and griot's library, for it is full of folklore, just as surely as it contains gallons of water. Baobab leaves, fruit, flowers, nuts, pods, bark, and oil are medicinal. It is often the only tree in its area, offering shelter from the elements and a point of visual and historical reference.

We left off in the last chapter with a friend's sacred water ritual, created in large part by orange, lemon, tangerine, live oak, and pine—trees that I hold sacred. Steadily, as we make our way through the wood, canopy to understory, north to south, we find that all types of trees have holistic medicines throughout. As I said earlier, it is very difficult to break trees down into categories.

With the fruit, berries, leaves, nuts, pods, beans, and berries spoken for, we turn toward the fruitful, the yield of the sacred wood. In this chapter, our focus is on tree barks, gums, resins, saps, and moss. Fittingly, many tree element saps are sacred, helping the user get in touch with divinity. Let's begin with a look at one of our more ancient trees, revered by the ancient Khemetians thousands of years ago: the acacia.

Acacia: Medicine Tree of the Savanna

The acacia (*Acacia nilotica*) was beloved of the ancient Khemetians, who linked it to deities, birth, death, the afterlife, and immortality. Some believed that gods were born underneath the goddess Saosis's acacia tree, north of Heliopolis. Horus is said to have emerged from within the acacia tree. With its association to sacred figures in the Khemetian cosmology, it is no wonder that acacia is considered healthy, magical, and linked to deity. Today, acacia trees continue to grow abundantly in Egypt.

>> *Acacia albida* is called *gozanga* in Ghana. A decoction of its bark is used as an anti-emetic and febrifuge. Steeped acacia bark is used as a bath or liniment for pneumonia.

>> A difficult labor may be soothed with a plain sitz bath in acacia, because of its demulcent qualities, or with the addition of shea butter for further lubricant.[1]

>> *Acacia farnesia*'s bark and leaf are used to make a lotion to cure ringworm and parasites that cause skin disease.

>> *Acacia hockii* (called *shittim* wood in Ghana) is decocted and prepared as a bath for leprosy. The trunk or branch wood smoke is used for fumigation.

>> The chewed bark, leaves, and pods of *Acacia nilotica var. tomentos* are prepared as a drink to cure scurvy. This type of acacia is also applied to ulcers or made into an ointment for exterior wounds.[2]

>> Gum of acacia consists primarily of arabin, a compound of arabic acid with calcium and varying amounts of magnesium and potassium salts, along with a trace of sugar.

>> Mucilage of acacia is nearly transparent, colorless, and viscid, with a faint though pleasant taste.

>> Senegal gum refers to acacia gathered from Sudan, Egypt, or Kordofan. Senegal gum possesses properties that make it superior and always preferred to other gums. *A. Senegal* (*Willd.*) comes from Senegambia in West Africa and the Upper Nile region of Eastern Africa.

>> Acacia resin is added to a "sacred blend" incense, lending the ability to connect the user with spirits that exist at high frequencies.

>> Gum acacia is a demulcent that sheathes inflamed interior surfaces. It is used to treat respiratory, digestive, and urinary tract ailments and also makes a useful treatment for diarrhea and dysentery.

>> Acacia has been known to combat the low stages of typhoid fever.

>> Gum acacia is administered as a mucilage (soaked and dissolved) called *Mucelago acaciae*.

>> Artists use gum acacia as a fluid medium, particularly with watercolors.

Creative Dragon's Blood

Dragon's blood, another multipurpose tree, comes from various species, including *Daemonorops draco* family *Palmae*, *Croton hibiscifolius*, *Calamus rotang* (East Indies, South and Central America), and *Pterocarpus draco* (East Indies and South America).

Its sap solidifies to a brilliant red resin. People often use dragon's blood ink from the resin of this African tree of the palm family to enhance their holistic lifestyle. It is used to form agreements and pacts and to write love letters. Dragon's blood is associated with passion, strength, vitality, and motivation, a carryover from the African perception of red as a power color. Dragon's blood is sold as an incense, a powder, and an ink. In West Africa, it is also consumed as an aphrodisiac.

The product called dragon's blood can come from any number of trees whose sap solidifies into red resinous chunks. Since it is such a natural curiosity—indeed, it is sold and used as a curio—many of the tree species from which it is derived are becoming overutilized, exploited crops that should be avoided. To circumvent this, some people simply buy red ink and add very small chunks of dragon's blood to symbolically imbue the ink with the tree's mystical power. For ecological reasons, this approach is preferable.

Camphor Tree (*Cinnamomum camphora*)

One of the African American cure-alls used when I was a child was camphorated oil. Camphor oil was added to a fixed oil and rubbed on the chest or around the nose. This method was used before companies started marketing ready-made preparations such as Vicks VapoRub. I also recall experiencing its rather acrid smell in mothballs. My mother was always placing them in our home; living in the wetlands sounds bucolic, and it looked that way, but at the same time the wetness was always worming into our home, sometimes leaving mildew in its wake. Mom put out the balls to override the smell of dampness, mold, and mildew that settled in, particularly during the infamous storms and heavy rains of a South Jersey spring to early summer season.

CAMPHORATED OIL

Camphorated oil doesn't have to be relegated to the annals of history. It can be made by adding a few drops of the essential oil to three tablespoons of melted aloe butter, shea butter, or mango butter. You can also add a drop or so of camphor oil to a handkerchief. Inhale the scent to clear nasal passages and sinuses at bedtime.

Camphor leaves have a clean-smelling aroma that is used as a sedative and calming agent in aromatherapy.

Camphor works on the central nervous system, treating convulsions, hysteria, and insomnia.

Camphor leaf is used to treat the uncomfortable symptoms of colds and flus and upper respiratory ailments. It is thought to be a good relief for rheumatism, muscle pains, and body aches.

WILD CAMPHOR TREE

Camphor of different types has been used on both sides of the Atlantic. Wild camphor (*Tarchonanthus camphorates*) was used in South Africa among the hunter/gatherer societies there. Today, several South African companies sell these "bush teas"—made of wildcrafted, organic indigenous herbs—internationally. Wild camphor offers many benefits. Khoi and San, two of the world's oldest cultures, have used these trees for thousands of years for camphor's soothing qualities in the following ways:

> Dried leaves of the wild camphor tree are used in ceremonies to anoint the body during rituals.

> Its leaves and seeds are used in fumigation. Camphor smoke treats rheumatism, headache, and insomnia.

> A tea made from wild camphor leaves relieves stomach ailments, asthma, anxiety, and heartburn.

> Wild camphor leaves also contain an insecticide that is used to deter lice and external parasites.

Cedar of Lebanon

Cedar trees (*Cedrus libani*) can grow to up to eighty feet, with a trunk up to three feet in diameter. The large, cone-bearing evergreen has a chunky trunk and a narrow pointy crown, becoming irregular and broad or flattened, spreading horizontally when allowed. Cedars grow in full sun, in well-drained, moist soil. The cones are three to four and a half inches long, barrel shaped, and tightly constructed.[3] As its name indicates, cedar of Lebanon

Wherever you live, you can cultivate a unique relationship with specific trees.

has a history in the Middle East. It is mentioned in the Bible and other ancient literature. The tree also grows in Nova Scotia and does especially well in the southeastern and northeastern United States.

Cedar is constantly in my life! At Paradise Lake, we had a spectacular trio of magnificent cedars at the edge of our property by the dock at the water's edge. This area of the yard was where as children we dried off after swimming, and ate the fish that Dad caught and grilled. We entertained suitors there. It was where I had my wedding and first baby shower. This trio of trees was clearly visible from the picture window of my bedroom and thus from my bed. They were the first trees I was able to observe from dusk to dawn, through varied weather conditions.

This is what I mean when I describe trees as markers. Wherever you live, you can cultivate a unique relationship with specific trees. Today, I have cedar at home in a different form—I use it for animal bedding, to create sachets, and to enhance my homemade incense. I use cedar oil in the same manner, adding a few drops to handmade floor wash to bring an outdoorsy scent inside.

Aromatic cedarwood timber and shavings were used to make Egyptian mummy cases, and they repel termites, moths, and other insects when used in linen chests, coat hangers, and closets.[4]

Balsamic resin of cedar is used in embalming, and it can be used in incense and cosmetics as well.

Essential oil from *C. L. atlantica*, steam distilled from the wood, is used in men's cologne. It is added to mosquito repellents, works as a leech repellent, and soothes anxiety and stress. Cedar oil is used to treat bronchial conditions and tuberculosis, and it inhibits tumor growth. (Warning: red cedar oil, a different type of cedar, acts as an aborifacient, and therefore it should be avoided by pregnant women or those trying to become pregnant.[5])

Cinnamon

The cinnamon tree (*Cinnamomum verum* J Presl; *Cinnamonium zeylanicum* Nees.) is a tropical evergreen tree famous for its aromatic bark, wood, and leaves.[6] It has a complex aroma, described variously as sweet, spicy, mellow, and rich. As the botanical Latin name suggests, the constituents in cinnamon are clearly related to the camphor tree (*Cinnamomum camphora*) previously discussed. The silk panicles of tiny malodorous cream flowers born in the summer eventually reveal purple berries. Cinnamon grows up to thirty feet and is grown in greenhouses elsewhere in well-drained, moisture retentive, sandy, yet fertile soil, under full sun or partial shade.

The ancient Khemetians and other cultures referred to cinnamon as cinnamomum and cassia. In contemporary culture, cassia, or cassia lignea, is used to describe the spice barks widely traded, called *Cinnamomum Cassia* (Nees) *Blume*. Cinnamon originated in Ceylon; it is native to East Africa, imported via the ancient Punt to coastal Somalia. The barks sold as cinnamon and cassia come from various parts of the diaspora, including Madagascar, Cape Verde Islands, Brazil, Cayenne, the West Indies, and Egypt. In some of these places it is highly productive, in particular Cayenne (French Guiana, South America). Cinnamon in trade is derived from various species of *Cinnamomum*.

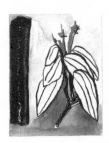

Historically in Khemet, cinnamon was not consumed orally but was used as a suppository to "cool the anus," presumably from hemorrhoids or lower colon disorders. The formula for this suppository consists of several other resins and tree materials, including juniper berries, frankincense and myrrh resins, and honey and other ingredients.[7]

Cinnamon is also the only spice used in mummification, presumably because it is a superb natural preservative. In mummification, cassia and cedar were sometimes used together, and mummies have been found filled with the two tree medicines.[8] Cinnamon continues to be a most useful herb in the kitchens and medicine kits of many cooks and herbalists.

MAGICAL AND SPIRITUAL USES OF CINNAMON

Cinnamon is used to energize hoodoo formulas in the following ways:

≫ To charge spaces with energy

≫ As a male aphrodisiac

≫ For scenting candles

≫ As a preservative in pomanders

≫ To add a bittersweet bite to incense

≫ As a scent preserver and aromatic in potpourri

It is also placed on altars, and outdoors at tree buttresses and roots, to invoke or petition specific deities.

Cinnamon is also of course used as a stimulating tea, or to flavor herbal medicines in various parts of Africa, as a digestive aid, and for adding flair to soul foods such as candied sweet potatoes or yams, sweet potato pie, in Caribbean drinks, smoothies, savory stews and dishes in West and North Africa, and curries in South Africa and Jamaica. It is also appreciated by herbalists for its antiseptic qualities.

Well, you get the point: there is a lot you can do with this herb bark, and our people have been working cinnamon in funerary rituals, ceremonies, magick, and medicine from the days of Punt and Khemet, and this work continues.

Resins, Gums, Saps, Moss, and Bark: The Gift to Urban Herbalists

I often get asked what you do if you are an urban herbalist without access to huge acreage for garden spaces, grounds, or forest gathering. The answer is twofold: first of all, *where there is a will, there is a way*. Cities and suburbs often include conservatories, botanic gardens, and forest preserves, yet you cannot necessarily harvest from these spaces. Still, you can enjoy the healing aura and akashic energy of trees in these spaces.

Urban gardeners: this chapter is a very important one for you. Resins in particular last for thousands of years. Yep, they'll outlive you and still perform admirably. Frankincense, found in a mummy believed to be thirty-five hundred years old, was retrieved, burned, and found to smell absolutely lovely, which means that it still contained its valuable essential oils. You can order frankincense or myrrh by the pound and store it in a clean, dry space for years. Gums and saps last six months to a year, as do barks and mosses.

Part of the issue with tender herbal parts, such as flowers and leaves, is that they break down, losing their medicinal quality rather quickly. This is not the case with the materials used in this chapter. The same holds true for tough wood, clove buds, or berry spices. The key is to obtain tree herbs from a reputable source and store them in an appropriate container in a clean, dry space that doesn't get a lot of light. It'll be good for many months or years of holistic healing, urban herbalists, as long as you decide to utilize African diasporic resins, gums, saps, moss, and barks like acacia, frankincense, myrrh, and cinnamon bark.

Magical Magnolia: Tree of Fidelity, Domesticity, and Good Health

Magnolia glauca, also called swamp laurel, swamp sassafras, and white bay, is an evergreen tree found in the Atlantic and Gulf Coast states. It is a breathtaking tree prominent in the southeastern United States, but magnolia also grows elsewhere; we even have a few young ones in our neighborhood, and it gets quite cold here. The tree has soft, leathery leaves, which are alternate, elliptical, glossy, and deep green on one side and pale underneath. Magnolia flowers revive the spirits and bring a warm, comforting atmosphere with them, inside the home or as a blooming specimen in the yard.

The creamy flowers are beloved by artists. They seem to soothe the mind and calm the spirit. One of the most beautiful renditions of the magnolia is an oil painting by American Hudson River School painter Martin Johnson Heade, painted in 1888.

The dried leaf is used in hoodoo as a natural amulet to instill monogamy and faithfulness in marital relationships. Magnolia leaf is put beneath the mattress and acts as a fidelity charm. It is also recommended as a newlywed luck charm tree.

In the garden, the tree ensures good luck and brightens the spirits of all who come near, especially during blooming season.

Magnolia bark is medicinal, an astringent, diaphoretic, febrifuge, and stimulant, and it also has tonic qualities. This tree medicine is also good for dyspepsia, dysentery, and various skin disorders, and it works as a douche for leukorrhoea. Magnolia bark has been used in folk medicine to treat tobacco and nicotine addiction, by aiding smoking cessation. This bark is gathered in the spring and summer. Whenever gathering bark, harvest sparingly with respect to the future growth of the tree.

Decoct magnolia bark using one teaspoon of bark to one cup of water. Take only a cup a day. For external treatments, simmer one tablespoon of bark to one pint of water for ten minutes, cool, and apply to skin with a cotton ball.[9]

Frankincense and Myrrh

The Khemetians as a culture loved trees, and nowhere is that more evident than with their preference for aromatic resins and fragrant herbs derived from all parts of the tree. Frankincense and myrrh are two naturally occurring incenses sacred to Khemetians, used in daily rites, funerary and mummification rituals, deity veneration, and celebration. The two trees enjoy kinship as members of the *Burseraceae* family, which consists of five hundred species in seventeen genera.[10]

These are two trees that work beautifully in concert, opening humans to the rich possibilities of higher consciousness of deity, spirit guides, and ascended masters.

The complementary combination of smoldering frankincense and myrrh evokes Anubis, Osiris, and Ra. When the resins are used as essential oil, they take on the feminine form, evoking Isis. Since Isis's attributes center on her protective abilities, she is thanked for security and abundance through the use of these two resins. Frankincense and myrrh are used as a special invocation.

In fact, frankincense in particular brings us parallel to spirit—it is a vehicle through which we can call the spirit home. Frankincense facilitates the ability to commune with various divine orders, including angelic spirits, carrying our love, prayers, and bids for protection to them. It helps keep our heart pure, and brings understanding and compassion, going so far as to heal the healer who suffers from guilt.[11] Carly Wall attributes some of frankincense's power to the chemical it gives off while burning, trahydroccanabinole, which in *The Scented Veil* she states is consciousness expanding. Wall also reminds us that frankincense was burned to free the ill of evil spirits, purging them from body and soul.[12]

Earthy yet spiritual, myrrh is intoxicating, deep, dark, and mysteriously forceful. I find it grounding, capable of easing the symptoms of cold and influenza. Myrrh is known to:

>> Heal

>> Strengthen

>> Ground

>> Purify

>> Uplift downward spirits

>> Relieve mental and physical anguish

>> Release past emotional blockages, letting creativity flow
   through the threshold of our consciousness.

These are two trees that work beautifully in concert, opening humans to the rich possibilities of higher consciousness of deity, spirit guides, and ascended masters. Serving as spiritual portals, frankincense and myrrh are capable of deepening spiritual connections. The resins are important to the celebration of holy days. This sacred duo is used for creating and maintaining consecrated space; gesticulating to the ancestors and spirits from the personal altar is possible with frankincense and myrrh.

Boswellia sacra and *Boswellia carterii*, known as *Beyo* and referred to as *olibanum*, is the classical frankincense distilled into essential oil. *Frank* means "free," *incense* means "lightning." The Arabic word for frankincense, *luban*, means "milk of the Arabs." Its earliest use is inscribed on the tomb of Queen Hatshepsut in the fifteenth century B.C.E. Somalia's commercial history began with incense; northern Somalia gained international significance through its incense trade. It is used locally as a fire starter, to deter snakes and scorpions, for purification, to perfume hair and clothing, in the purses of Arab women as solid perfume, as incense, and in holy ointments. It is even used in a cola soft drink. *Beyo* is still imported primarily from

Somalia (ancient Punt), East Africa. It also grows around the horn of Africa and in the Hadhramaut region of Yemen and Oman. In Ghana, frankincense is referred to as "incense tree" or *kabona,* and it comes from *Boswellia dalzielii.* Fresh *kabona* bark is chewed as an emetic. Insecticide is made from burning frankincense resins. Frankincense is chewed as an emetic to relieve symptoms of palpitation. A bath created from a decoction of frankincense is used to treat rheumatism.[13]

Urged on by my friend Mark Ambrose, former owner of Scents of Earth, whom I call the poet laureate of fragrance, I got into frankincense in its pure and highest forms about five years ago. I like to experiment with different types from various regions. I burn it, ground with a small portion of ground myrrh. The essential oil also works very well as an astringent for troubled skin. It is a good addition to natural soap and cosmetics. Frankincense is the pathway to spiritual enlightenment, used in the home, studio, and worship environment. It is enjoyed in the African diaspora, particularly in the United States and parts of the Caribbean, as incense and anointment oil.

Maydi is the top grade of medicinal frankincense. Used as a chewing product in Saudi Arabia, *maydi* comes in seven grades, the highest two being preferred. *Mushaad* and *mujaarwal,* numbers one and two, respectively, are close to transparent, sold as quite large and unbroken pieces. *Maydi* that survives shipment abroad is usually the smaller, opaque, lower-grade types.

MYRRH: FROM ANCIENT AFRICA TO THE PRESENT

Just as with frankincense, the highest grades of myrrh (*Commiphora myrrh* and *C. abyssynia*) still come from Somalia and Ethiopia.

African practitioners of many paths and religions use myrrh spiritually. Heliopolis myrrh was burned at noon to invoke and praise the ancient Egyptian sun god Ra. Myrrh is also burned to honor the Egyptian moon goddess Isis. Ghanaians fumigate clothing with the fragrant smoke of burning myrrh wood. Swahili speakers use frankincense as a diuretic. The bark of myrrh tree is used as a tonic in East Africa.[14]

British herbalist Anne McIntyre suggests frankincense to heal many conditions, including respiratory infections, catarrh, laryngitis, asthma, fevers, scars, sores, and wounds. Myrrh is a stimulant, carminative, vulnerary, expectorant, antiseptic, antiviral, and detoxifier. It is useful for bronchitis, asthma, colds, indigestion, and inflammation.[15]

You'll find myrrh on your health food store shelves in mouthwash or toothpaste, to deter gingivitis, periodontal disease, mouth ulcers, and toothache. Tom's Natural Toothpaste and Mouthwash features myrrh as a dentifrice. I have decocted myrrh resin quickly and easily in my kitchen and used it for my children's toothaches and sore throats with a cold. The versatile resin is also added to lotions, potpourri, perfumery, soap, baths, and food (approved by FDA) as a preservative of scent.

The resins are pounded to a usable size with a mortar and pestle and burned over charcoal to create incense. There should be two parts frankincense, which is sweet, light, and airy, to one part myrrh, which is the deep, earthy base note. This combination helps create a highly charged, bright spiritual vibration.

Pau D'arco: Divine Bark

Pau d'arco (*Tabebruiae impeliginosa*) is native to the Central and South American rainforests. The tree has bright green, oval-shaped leaves with thick golden seams, and cut designs resembling mosaic in each serrated leaf. The tree blooms with clusters of dangling purple trumpet-shaped flowers. Early medicine men peeled the tree's bark in long strips. They separated the outer bark from the purple inner bark to make tea, which was considered a panacea for centuries.

It is called "divine bark" in Brazil, Mexico, Argentina, and the Bahamas, where it is considered a cure-all. Pau d'arco's divinity stems from the fact that it attracts alpha rays, which exert a positive electrical charge on human cells, since crystalline oxygen is trapped in its inner bark.

Pau d'arco contains vitamins A, B complex, and C and minerals iron, calcium, selenium, magnesium, manganese, zinc, phosphorous, potassium, and sodium. It contains flavonoids, alkaloids, quinines, and saponins. The antitumor agent it contains, lapachol, inhibits cancer growth and lymph congestion.[16] Known uses of pau d'arco include:

≫ Antibiotic

≫ Antibacterial

≫ Antimicrobial

≫ Antifungal

≫ Anti-tumor

≫ Immune system stimulant

≫ Disease fighter

≫ Mucous congestion

≫ For psoriasis, eczema, ringworm, and scabies

≫ Throat, mouth, and gums show improvement with pau d'arco tea, either taken internally or used as a rinse.

In Brazil, pau d'arco is also used for prostatitis, gonorrhea, gastric intestinal disorders, and respiratory ailments. In the Bahamas, pau d'arco bark decoction is used to treat backache, gonorrhea, toothache, lack of sexual desire (aphrodisiac), and incontinence. [17]

I have used it to replenish the strength of people who have severe illnesses, such as HIV/AIDS and cancer, as well as to treat the symptoms of transient illnesses such as cold and influenza.

The chemical constituents naphthaquinones, found in pau d'arco bark, have substantial antifungal properties validated by laboratory tests. This chemical group also has the ability to fight cancer. Pau d'arco bark has killed lung cancer cells in laboratory tests, reducing the rate of lung tumor growth in mice. I have experienced this result with my own father, but I did not give him massive doses, nor did I give capsules. Instead, we used the natural bark as a decoction. The National Cancer Institute agrees: the whole bark has no known side effects. Unrefined pau d'arco bark is safer than taking extracts of the active ingredients.[18] The National Cancer Institute has stated that to be effective the bark needs to be taken in such large doses as to render it toxic for positive effects to occur. The American Cancer Society does not recommend pau d'arco as an alternative treatment for cancer until more evidence becomes available.[19]

I have found that as a complimentary, alternative medicine (CAM), where it is used in moderate doses in conjunction with pharmaceutical biomedicines, it offered relief. When patients say they don't want drugs, that they would rather use herbs, it is important to realize that herbs contain drugs and therefore must be used as carefully as pharmaceuticals. Pau d'arco is a promising herb with a venerable history among traditional American and African Caribbean people that the medical establishment

---

Extracting Pau D'arco

Decoct 2 tablespoons of dried pau d'arco bark in 10 ounces of simmering water, covered, over medium heat for 20 minutes. Remove from heat. Let cool for 10 minutes. Strain through a sieve to remove the bark. Sweeten if desired with honey. Sip. Drink no more than 2 cups per day.

has not quite figured out yet. It is always useful for you to read the available literature. Keep up with the latest laboratory testing and scientific findings regarding tree medicines of choice, deciding from there how to proceed.

While herbal medicines are criticized by the establishment or hyped by the media, whatever the mood of the day may be, herbalists stay attuned to the folk wisdom of traditional people, keeping aware of what they have used effectively for hundreds of years. As contemporary practitioners, we also read literature from places such as the German E Commission and the Herb Research Society.

White Willow

Aspirin is one of those wonder drugs, simple and homey. Many have grown up hearing "Take two aspirin and call me in the morning." As close to an American cure-all as we are likely to get, the medicine in aspirin comes from the willow tree (*Salix alba*). It hasn't been until very recently that the scientific community has more fully understood and appreciated the healing impact of willow.

White willow grows in north Africa, central Asia, Europe, and the northeastern United States. It has rough gray bark, and grows to seventy-five feet, though it is also maintained as a shrub. White willow is a balancing herb associated with magic, earth-based spirituality, and healing. It is a tree that holds tremendous healing potential.

In the West, no magical herbalist's property is complete without the willow, whether it is the tree, a bough, or a wreath. Willow invokes healing energy, from its sympathetic bearing to its preferred habitat near the water's edge. In or near the water is considered otherworldly in West African traditional paths, a site followers of African-inspired spirituality also appreciate.

> **Willow Tea**
>
> Infuse 1 to 3 teaspoons of willow bark in cold water for from 2 to 5 hours. Only 1 cup per day is recommended.[20]

On the Yoruba-derived *Ifa* path, orisha Obatala addresses the white fluids of the body, called *funfun*. These white or colorless fluids are key to the healer's oeuvre, containers of *ashe*. White willow is one of Obatala's healing herbs, used to petition his wisdom and as an offering to his wise spirit.

For over two thousand years, white willow has been used to alleviate pain. It contains salicin, an aspirinlike medicine that helps reduce inflammation. Traditionally, willow has been used to treat rheumatism, internal bleeding, gum and tonsil inflammation, and eruptions, sores, burns, and wounds.

Willow bark is collected with respect and reverence in the spring, followed by a prayer of appreciation.

Oak Moss

Grounding and maintaining a connection to the earth should be a daily practice of the healer and those seeking wellness. It is important to seek out and keep a small portion of oak moss (*Evernia prunastri*) on hand at all times.

The thalli of oak moss are short and bushy and grow together on the bark to form clumps, which resemble deer antlers. The deer's gentle spirit is greatly respected in Africa, and its horns are used to carry *ashe* medicine. Oak moss's resemblance to deer antlers is welcomed in diasporic and African-inspired practices. Oak moss is a lovely and earthy sage green color, described as grayish green to white. Its distinct and complex odor is woodsy, sharp, or slightly sweet.

Oak moss is a type of lichen found in many mountainous temperate forests throughout the northern hemisphere. Oak moss grows on the trunks and branches of oak trees, but also on the bark of other deciduous and coniferous trees, such as fir and pine. The oak moss growing on pines has more of a pronounced turpentine aroma.

Oak moss is an herb I maintain close contact with. I use it a great deal in perfumery. It is a preferred vehicle for holding the scents of essential oils in potpourris and sachets, which are great ways to infuse the home with forest energy. According to aromatherapy and spirituality expert Dr. Valerie Ann Worwood in *The Fragrant Heavens*, oak moss is spiritually grounding, connecting humans to the earth.[21]

From Slave Wood to Freedom Herb: Secretive Quassia

Quassia (*Picraena excelsa L*), pronounced kwosh-uh, is a West Indian and South American tree. Jamaican quassia is *Picrasma excelsa*. The Jamaican type is taller than the Surinamese, Brazilian, or West Indian type. It also grows in French Guiana, the islands of Dominica, Martinique, St. Lucia, St. Vincent, and Barbados. The name given by the founder of the genus was *Carib simarouba*. The tree grows to sixty feet tall or more, with many long, crooked branches covered in smooth, grayish bark. Its large leaves are nine to twelve inches long. The flowers grow in small clusters with thick, off-white petals. Quassia bark is usually found in pieces several feet long. The roots are long, horizontal, and creeping. It is odorless and difficult to powder. It is frequently imported from Jamaica in bales.

The secret of quassia is how it came to our knowledge. It is also called "slave wood," which provides an important clue. An enslaved person named Quassi held the secret to this tree's medicine from his native Suriname for quite a while. Eventually, he sold the secret to Rolander, a Swede, in around 1756. Some accounts say the secret medicine held in the tree was revealed from the dream realm and shared with Quassi; this is a recurring theme in African and African diaporic healing, because dreams are highly regarded for their ability to provide prophetic signs. White doctors looked on as Quassi "doctored" people of all races, readily reducing what would have been a deadly fever. He gave freely, but did not want to reveal what was contained within the potion.

In the end, he sold the recipe; some accounts say that it was for a large sum of money, while others say that it was in exchange for his freedom. This practice, trading herbal knowledge for emancipation, has also been noted as a part of our history.[22] Quassia was very important as a cure for dysentery. In 1713, it was sent to France. Between 1718 and 1725, an epidemic flu prevailed in France, which resisted all the usual medicines. Quassia was tried, and it was very successful.

The so-called slave wood became sought-after medicine in Europe during the eighteenth century. It is still used by West Indians, and it was a time-honored European cure for fever, malaria, snakebite, dysentery, dyspepsia, sexually transmitted diseases, rheumatism, alcoholism and other addictions, and intestinal worms and cancer.

Quassia is a pure bitter, once sold in wooden cups made of the tree. Water extracts and dilutes quassia readily, making this a very sensible eco-package. Quassia was used to discourage thumb sucking. As an intense bitter, it is used as a substitute for hops in making beer. It is used in tonics and for wine making.

Quassia contains a bitter identical to quassin (a resinous and volatile oil), malic acid, gallic acid, and small amounts of other constituents. It is used as a restorative for lost tone of the intestines. It also promotes cleansing and purging secretions, treats insomnia, kills lice in the hair of children, and is used as a pesticide. It is sometimes set out in saucers as an infusion and used to kill flies, mealy bugs, and gnats.

Most important, quassia contains medicine that eases the later stages of dysentery, when the stomach is not affected. This is helpful to people who prefer forest remedies, and it is useful to those who have little access to reliable pharmaceuticals.

Wild Cherry

The wild cherry (*Prunus serotina*), an aromatic tree with a tall trunk, oblong crown, numerous white flowers, and small black cherries, is one of North America's most useful trees. The pounded leaf and bark releases an aroma similar to cherry, and is a bitter like quassia. Wild cherry, or choke cherry as it is also called, grows widely in North America, therefore it can be safely wildcrafted. It is one of our largest, most significant trees for lumber, paneling, wood handles, and other wood products.

Wild cherry bark yields a famed folk remedy, cherry cough syrup, and, when compounded with horehound, cherry cough drops. We have also used this tree historically to yield fruit wine, jam, and jellies. This was one of the first medicinal trees I was exposed to, largely because, visioning through the portal, I saw that it could help strengthen or at least treat my mother's asthmatic condition and her coughing. I learned of wild cherry's useful medicines in one of the first widely available herbalist's guides, Jethro Kloss's *Back to Eden*, and then searched my environment to locate the tree and experiment with its fruit and bark. We have so much information available to us in America, in the Internet information age, but, more powerful than simply reading, measuring ingredients, or adhering to what others have done, our own touch, sight, smell, and extrasensory experience—the basis of African traditional medicine—is still our best guide to learning the full potential of the medicines covered in this book.

The Gullah people of Georgia's and South Carolina's sea coast and islands have many recorded folk remedies for various tree medicines and other herbs. The Gullah use a decoction of wild cherry bark, served cold, to immediately stop menstrual flow.

They also make a cough syrup of cherry and hickory bark, along with horehound leaves and sugar, to treat the symptoms of colds, such as hoarseness and sore throat.[23]

Bark, gum, saps, and resins have been used by Africans for over three thousand years. Evidence remains inside mummies' bodies and in the choice materials of their cases, and is found in ancient material medica. These parts of the tree, as well as lichen and moss, continue to be important in the holistic medicine of Africa and the New World. Critical to understanding our past as healers, tree medicines continue to be instrumental to our future as a holistically healthy culture. One of the most fascinating aspects of barks, gums, saps, resins, and mosses is that they strike an equal chord in our sacred life as in the mundane.

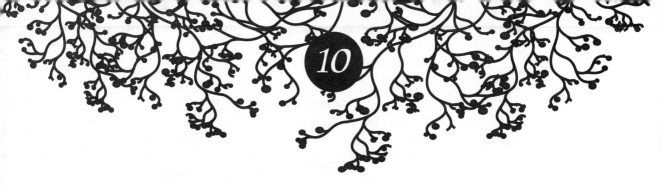

Very Important Palms

VIPS OF THE TRANSATLANTIC TREE WORLD

She does not know her beauty
She thinks her brown body
Has no glory.
If she could dance naked,
Under palm trees
And see her image in the river
She would know.
But there are no palm trees on the street,
And dishwater gives back no images.
    —bell hooks, "Sisters of the Yam"[1]

VIPs of the African Tree World

Palms are a highly prized holistic health tree, originally coming from Asia[2] but flourishing now in Africa and the diaspora, in forests, rainforest canopy, and the Amazon. They yield precious oil, skin and hair care, nutrition, mythology, divination, and spirituality and are emblems of faith. There are about 225 genera, with 2,650 species of palm—they are everywhere and into everything. The most used palms in your kitchen are probably coconut and palm oil. Palm is so important to the tree world that a standard leaf shape—palmate, which you've heard mentioned in these pages on many occasions, is derived from the shape of the palm leaf.

Palmate-leaved palms are incidentally the hardest of the bunch. The root word *palm* is also used to describe an acidic quality in plants—palmic acid is a common and essential fatty acid. Not to go on and on, but put simply, palms are so vital to African diasporic life that I venture to call them *the* VIPs: Very Important Palms.

The palm is the inside of our hand you offer peacefully to greet others, raising it at school in affirmation to say, "Yes, I'm here; I exist"—this same palm shape is a palmate leaf as it exists in nature.

I'm not sure where soapmaking would be at all were it not for palm. The chief vegetable oils used in soapmaking, for many of those "vegetarian" and "organic" natural products making waves on the marketplace, are created in large part from none other than two oils of the palm family, which we will discuss in a bit, palms and coconut. This chapter highlights:

>> Palm oil's use in health and beauty beyond soapmaking; the finest replaces cocoa butter as a chocolate additive and is used in cosmetics, confections, baking, and cooking.

>> Babassu as a symbol of sustainability and economic parity; its international presence is owed to indigenous American women who brought together politics, mythology, and plants.

>> Murumuru as a tree of folklore, food, and holistic health.

>> Acai as a superfood, with an abundance of healing energy and antioxidants.

>> Saw palmetto, once mainly primarily Seminole, Lumbee, and Gullah medicine, as now enjoyed by the whole world, providing good tree medicine for men's health.

>> Cork, rattan, and carnauba wax as clear and present in our domestic lives within the home; all come from palm trees.

>> Wine and other bottle seals—created from cork.

>> Bulletin boards—created from cork.

>> Chairs, tables, containers, and basketry—made from rattan.

>> Vegan furniture wax—falls from none other than the carnauba tree.

CARNAUBA

A fabulous vegetable wax is obtained by shaking the carnauba tree (*Copernicia prunifera*), also called the wax palm tree. This wax is suitable for vegans who do not use beeswax, and it is a fitting replacement for beeswax in some cosmetic formulations. Carnauba wax is used commercially to make vinyl records, candles, and floor and fine furniture wax. The young seeds from kernels are edible.

COQUILLA NUT

"What's that around your neck?" I often hear. "Is it (gulp) ivory?" "Heck no!" is all I can say. "It's coquilla nut," one of forty kinds of different palms found in Brazil.

Coquilla nut (*Attalea funifera*) resembles ivory, and it can be used as a substitute for it because it shares ivory's mellow, warm, off-white color and makes a great hard surface to carve with intricate shapes and patterns. The nut, which is being used in several "save the rainforest" programs, has an especially hard shell covering its four-inch dark frame. This cruelty-free substitute for ivory is also sustainable. Coquilla nut is used to make buttons, doorknobs, and jewelry. Similar species to coquilla nut are used to create broom and brush handles.

Another palm producing a hard nut, the ivory palm, or elephant plant (*Phytele phas*), has large hard seeds that are used to make billiard balls. This tree provides another cruelty-free ivory substitute.

CORK PALM

Cork palm (*Microcycas calocoma*) is in the cycad family, and, like several cycads, it is considered a living fossil. It grows in the Pinar del Rio region of Vinales Valley, an area that dates back three hundred million years. The rare Cuban prehistoric tree began life during the Cretaceous Period and is considered a valuable link to the history of plant life on earth. UNESCO has declared the Cork Palm a World Heritage. It is the type of plant that speaks to our akashic self by providing spiritual commune with the ancient natural world and our place within it.

Other useful corks grow and are commercially harvested in Portugal, a country that has an important connection to African cultures, particularly through slavery. Corks also grow elsewhere in the Mediterranean.

PALMYRA PALM

An eighty-foot tree from tropical Africa, the palmyra palm (*Borassus flabellifer*) also grows in Asia. Palmyra palm supplies durable wood. Its leaves are used for thatching roofs and to make writing paper. Palmyra palm leaves are also used for making mats, bags, baskets, umbrellas, and many more utilitarian objects.

The tender seeds of palmyra are soft, sweet, gelatinous, and pulpy, with little liquid, and they are relished during hot summer months because they yield good jelly. Palmyra pulp gradually hardens into a bony kernel, which develops into a fibrous coat and yields a cream-colored substance with the consistency of cheese and a pleasant taste. Palmyra sap with sugar makes a treat called *jaggery*; it is distilled to make toddy.[3] Seedlings of palmyra send out tender edible shoots two to three inches long and supply the foundation for starchy flour.

PEACH PALM

Peach palm (*Pupunha, pejibaye, Bactris, gasipaes, syn. Guilielma gasipaes*) has a growing range from Central America to Ecuador, where it is an important food crop. The fruit weighs up to twenty-five pounds and contains a high percentage of oil. Peach palms are used extensively, especially in Costa Rica, where their hearts (heart of palm) are processed, eaten as an appetizer, in salads or alone, and are a popular export. I do not condone the consumption of hearts of palm because harvesting them kills the tree.

RATTAN

Climbing palms (*Calamus spp*) belong to several genera from West Africa. There are 370 species of calamus, which is also called rattan cane.[4] The stems and leaves are barbed with vicious curving spines that hook onto other plants. The inner part of the shoots can be eaten. The fibers make a tough and reliable material for furniture.

CALAMUS ROOT

Pulverized, or cut and sifted, calamus root is beloved by herbalists, hoodoos, and rootworkers. Calamus root has a subtle earthen smell, and it is used as a scent and as a botanical preservative for homemade potpourri and other herbal blends such as botanical powders and sachets. In hoodoo, calamus root is respected as an aphrodisiac, noted for its ability to draw love.

WINE PALM

Palm wine is tapped from the male flowers of the wine palm (*Raphia hookeri*), and the trees are typically felled once tapped, which requires the consideration of a more sustainable solution and treatment for the revered tree. They can be left standing, but the tree still dies, like heart palms, when harvested.[5] Palm wine contains natural yeast, so its residue is used for baking. Its central shoot is called palm cabbage. The midrib of wine palm is used to create brooms, and the fronds supply fencing and roofing material.

The Metaphysical Dimensions of Palm

Ash Wednesday is the first day of Lent; the ashes are a somber reminder to con-template spiritual redirection. The ashes used in the Catholic church ceremony to mark a cross on the forehead come from burning the palms that are distrib-uted on Palm Sunday (last Sunday before Easter) the year before. The palms are symbolic of the palms that were thrown in the path of Jesus as he entered Jerusalem for his crucifixion. So, as with it all, is a cycle: celebrate death, for in death comes new life.

—Jannette Giles-Hypes, recovering Catholic and freethinker

The spiritual and metaphysical properties of the palm cross many cultures. In spiritual practice, the palm tree aids ritual and marks ceremony while symboli-cally enriching faith. The African love of mythology and folklore weaves the palm into both sacred and mundane life. Yet another purpose of the palm is as an oracle. Beginning with a quote from my dear friend Jannette, a fellow herbalist, this section of this chapter gives voice to these varied aspects of the mighty palm.

SACRED PALM NUT OF IFA

In West Africa's *Ifa* path, the palm nut is sacred to the almighty orisha Orunmila. Devotees use sacred palm nuts with *babalawo* during readings, or alone for prayer. Only a fragment of its magical importance and spiritual symbolism has been revealed to those uninitiated. Here is a brief description of the workings of the sacred palm nut as we know it.

First of all, it is good to visualize the roots of palms. They are so strong that they hang on to fragile sandy shores, often providing *Sacred palm is feared and respected.*

the only tree cover for humans, plants, and animals. This is because they not only have tensile strength, but they are also great energy conduits.[6] Our cultural roots rely heavily on palm for food, sustenance, and shelter. They are the site of petition and offering, and are used in divination because of their heavy symbolism.

This section primarily discusses the palm nuts of Ifa, *ekuro Ifa* or *Ikin Ifa*. These nuts are different from ordinary palm nuts. (Ordinary palm nut is called *ekuro* and comes from the oil palm.) The multipurpose palm nut is *Ikin Ifa*. Sacred palm is feared and respected. It is from *Elaeis idolatrica* and is used almost exclusively in ritual, hence its Latin name *E. idolatrica*. The *Ikin Ifa* tree is branched. Its nut has four eyes or more, and oil overflows from its black cast iron pot, causing a grease fire rather rapidly. Because of its tendency to overflow from its sacred container, the black pot that is likened to a womb, it has a great deal of mysticism attached to it. The branches, called *ori* or head, can have as many as sixteen eyes. *Ikin Ifa* are shiny black, beautiful, sumptuous, and sensual—a promising container of *dudu awo*.

Palm's rituals are varied; one is to collect young palm fronds that stand erect (a positive symbol) encircling the *ori* of the tree to make wine or oil used in ritual. These same types of fronds are used to set apart sacred groves (as discussed earlier). The frond's presence indicates divinity or spirit. The blackness held within represents sacred *awo*.[7]

> *Every part of community life is put* *before* babalawo *through his gift of divining with* Ikin Ifa.

A central object to *Ifa*, *Ikin Ifa* are presented to each *babalawo* when his training is completed. Every part of community life is put before *babalawo* through his gift of divining with *Ikin Ifa*. By gaining an understanding of *Ikin Ifa*, knowledge is gained of the divine nature of the palm tree itself. Sixteen black palm nuts at the heart of *Ifa* ritual are kept in their special container when not used for divination.

Dudu Osun: The Hidden Medicine

One of the founding principles of Yoruba medicine is the separation of what is hidden from what is revealed. Much of the "hidden" is spiritual, at the level of the soul or the inner workings of the body. The "revealed" is everything we can observe on the exterior, with some of the focus on male and female bodily fluids. As I have mentioned, *dudu* is Yoruban healer terminology for black. Black is one of three significant color symbols; the others are red (blood and earth) and white (sperm and spirituality). The Yoruba notion of black includes green and blue, colors of nature. As you can imagine, it is also used to describe the people of African descent. *Dudu*

Dudu osun makes use of all parts of trees and plants, making it ecological. It also helps otherwise fragile incomes, mostly of rural African women, lending to a successful economic botany enterprise, which in turn contribute to the overall health of the community.

is soil's color, and it represents the concept of burial as well as planting seeds. Black represents the skin as a container of soul, and the water lies beneath it—*dudu* is the interior of the self and how we should tend to it.

Tending to the skin is emphasized in African healing because skin is a strong indicator of health. Medicinal soaps are a very important method of herbal healing. In Yoruba medicine, soap is called *ose*. One of West Africa's great healing medicines is *dudu osun*, commonly called black soap in the United States. To this day, its ingredients and preparation remain a well-kept secret. We do know that its rich black color is created through the use of the unique herbal preparation technique called *etu* ("burnt medicine"), wherein the ingredients are slowly charred, and which relies on the potash of numerous indigenous tree leaves. *Dudu osun* features palm, a highly prized holistic health tree, used in cooking, beauty, healthcare, storytelling, and divination.

In *dudu osun,* palm oil is saponified. It contains *ashe*, liquid medicine with a healing force, from lime and lemon and other indigenous herbs. While the exact recipe for the medicine within *dudu osun* stays hidden, its healing benefits have long been revealed.

Dudu osun is used to treat skin and scalp irritations including eczema, seborrhea, psoriasis, itching, burning, flaking, wounds, acne, dandruff, boils, lesions, and leprosy. It is used as a soap, shampoo, and conditioner. While we can buy proprietary blends of the soap base to make something akin to it, for now, the truth about *dudu osun* is wrapped in the cloak of secrecy.

The palm is associated with Sonponno in the spiritual beliefs of *Ifa*. This is a most feared orisha associated with smallpox, whipping winds, skin diseases, and epidemics. Palm wine, called *emu*, keeps Sonponno away. Here are a few other ways palm is used spiritually and metaphysically:

A beautiful woman in African art is presented as well coiffed, with an elegant long neck and shiny lustrous skin.

Many tree leaves and barks are burned, producing potash used in soapmaking.

>> A broom made from the midribs of the palm frond is used to symbolize smallpox epidemics. Sometimes these brooms are bewitched to make a bad person, usually a thief, tire himself or herself by sweeping until he or she passes out. A palm frond broom is smeared with red camwood and kept in the smallpox victim's room.

>> During a smallpox epidemic, people drink palm wine to chase that particular orisha away.

>> Palm wine is splashed about the yard, courtyard, or verandah as a libation to keep Sonponno away.

>> Obatala, on the other hand, is a white orisha who likes to consume white things, so he drinks raffia palm called *oli oguro*.

>> Palm oil is a spiritual antidote to smallpox as well.

>> Palm kernel oil, called *adin*, is an offering to Sonponno, used to tease and annoy him so he will go away, curing the disease.

>> Palm wine is associated with revelation, which destroys internal order.[8]

>> *Babalawo* uses both palm nuts as tools of divination.

Raffia Palm

Raffia palm is used in ceremonial costuming for seasonal ritual, with the purpose of arbitrating with the spirits of the sacred wood. Not to make light of the hundreds of cultures using palm in ritual or ceremony, here is a small sampling of a few African groups and the ways they use raffia to illustrate the point.

ZAIRE'S KUBA

Kuba is the name given to about seventeen neighboring ethnic groups of the western Kasai region of south-central Zaire, also known as Kuba Kingdom, though it consists of numerous chiefdoms.[9] Kuba are renowned for their ability to transform raffia into exquisite cloth known as Kuba cloth. The people also fabricate raw forest materials, such as *makadi* (leaflets from a palm tree), using them to create costumes.

BOMA OF NIGERIA

Boma clan of Ijo village, Rivers State, Nigeria, has a time of the year when costumed performers wear a mask of natural raffia and other forest material. The performer moves from one end of the town to another like a gigantic broom, sweeping the community clean of its annual buildup of pollution, whether physical or metaphysical.

DAN OF CÔTE D'IVOIRE

Dan people of Côte d'Ivoire have their own masks and costumes, which usually feature grass such as raffia to indicate forest power. *Wo Puh Gle* is a talking entertainer, while *Yeh to Gle* is an authority figure. Go Society has a mask and costume called *Ga Wree Wree*. *Ga Wree Wree* is fierce symbol of powers that lurk within the forest. This mask contains leopard teeth and is embellished with raffia. It is primarily red, as red is the quintessential power color of life force and blood. The huge bell-shaped skirt of the costume is made entirely of raffia. The *Ga Wree Wree* performer walks or sits immersed in the grassy folds of the skirt. *Ga Wree Wree* is a creature that oversees and then passes judgment on the activities of the community, according to custom.

As a representative of "wild spirit," these ritual- and ceremony-bound outfits highlight a few of the numerous ways raffia palm is used to arbitrate with and represent the spirit of the sacred wood.

Melding of the Phoenix and the Palm: Meet the Date Palm

The phoenix is a mythic animal and spiritual omen. You won't be surprised, considering the longevity and powerful cultural impact this birdlike spirit being has cast over Africa, beginning in Khemet, to find that its name is lent to an important palm tree.

The botanical name of date palm, *Phoenix dactylifera L.*, is derived from a Phoenician word, *phoenix*, which means "date palm," and *dactylifera*, a derivative of the Greek word *daktulos*, which means finger, describing the fruit's shape.[10] What we consider fruit is an inflorescence, growing between the leaves and hanging out from the sides of the tree.

A couple of other sources refer to its botanical name in connection to the Egyptian phoenix, which lived to be five hundred years old, casting itself into a fire from which it arises fully renewed.[11] This analogy to the date palm, which can also renew itself after significant fire damage, makes sense of the spirit bird and date palm sharing a botanical name, whereas *dactylifera* originates from Hebrew, *dachel*, a descriptor for the fruit's shape.[12]

Date palm is an angiosperm called *Monocotyledones*; the *Palmaceae*, the family to which it belongs, consists of about two hundred genera and fifteen hundred species. Phoenix (*Coryphoideae phoeniceae*) is a genus containing about a dozen species, all native to tropical or subtropical regions of Africa or southern Asia, including *Phoenix dactylifera* L.[13]

In modern Egyptian Arabic the tree is called *nahl* and the fruit is *balol*.

Like the mythology and folklore that sprang up around the phoenix, the date palm has also grown in Egypt since prehistoric times, and it is still a predominate feature of Nile Valley landscape. Here are some of its uses:

≫ Dates are distilled for various aperitifs and liquors.

≫ The insides of the top of the date palm trunk are edible and taste like celery.

≫ Soldiers once ate its fruit in Greece, and eat it now in Iraq.

≫ Dates are so coveted that they were used as currency to pay workers in Egypt.

≫ During classical pharaonic eras of ancient Egypt, wine was made from palm dates and sweetened with honey.

≫ Date palm wine was used during ceremonies and ritual during mummification. It was used to wash the bodies of mummies.

≫ The fruits were and still are pressed into blocks and hung on strings.

≫ Date wood is used for roofing, the fibers for basketry, and the leaves for brushes and ropes.

≫ Date juice was a major sweetener in the days before sugar beet and sugar cane.

Today, health-conscious people trying to reduce sugar consumption—and its ecological implications—are returning to the date's sweet quality, using it as a sweetener in baked goods, foods, drinks, and smoothies. The fruits are eaten fresh or dried. High in fiber and energy, dates are one of my favorite healthy snacks. Dates are used herbally in several herbal treatments: infusions, potions, suppositories, unguents, and poultices. Dates are also mashed, infused, and used to create poultices which fill the nostrils to cure sneezing fits, or are placed on the legs to reduce swelling.[14]

The Big Three: Africa's Fabulous Oil Palms

AFRICAN PALM

Palm oil is the quintessential West African oil, used commercially and in house-holds to make soap, to cook with, and to create healing balms. African palm (*Elaeis guineensis*) originated in Africa and is now cultivated throughout the tropics. This tree flourishes in Nigeria, a major producer of palm oil, as well as in Côte d'Ivoire, Ghana, Benin Republic, and Togo.[15] Nigeria is by far the most important source of edible palm oil. The nuts are encased in a fibrous covering, containing three vari-eties. Varieties are distinguished by the seed color, orange or black. Orange seeds yield the finest oil, but have small kernels. Brazilians call orange palm oil *dende*. Oth-ers have less oil but larger nuts, which are roasted and eaten. Numerous Brazilian and West African dishes contain *dende*. The reddish-orange palm oil contains beta-carotene, a noted antioxidant and precursor to vitamin A. High grades of palm oil are added to chocolate, replacing the cocoa butter additive. Some facts about palm oil:

- Palm kernel is 50 percent oil.
- Palm kernel oil is used in confections, ice cream, and shortening.
- Fruits of the palm are used to make a soup called *abenkwan*.[16]
- It is expensive, due to its high demand; the oil is vital for African soapmaking.
- Palm oil is grown in rural areas, in the country, and in the forest.
- Palm kernel oil is associated more with urban locales.

ARGAN PALM

Argan (*Medemia argun, Wurltemb. ex Mart*), is a fan palm but its stem is not branched. It has an ellipsoid edible fruit of a deep purple color, with yellow flesh. The argan tree grows sparsely in the Sudan. In ancient Egypt, it was a garden tree. Fruits of the argan have been found in burials of the fifth dynasty.[17]

Argan oil comes from *Argania spinosa*. It is rich in antioxidants, flavonoids, and tocopherols. This oil contains a high percentage of polyphenols and almost double the amount of tocopherols in olive oil. The tree is native to southwestern Morocco, near Agadir. The plum-sized fruits are eaten by goats that climb the trees—women once harvested the fruits from goat droppings. Nowadays, modern technology has eliminated this process for the most part. The kernels are striped off the fruit by machine and cold pressed to express the oil. Argan oil has a specific aroma and is considered a gourmet's necessity in Moroccan cooking. It is also used in hair conditioners and soap.

COCONUT

Coconut (*Cocos nucifera*) is useful, practical, and economical—a wonderful gift of the palm world. It is a major African cash crop, benefiting the economies of Ghana, Côte d'Ivoire, Kenya, Nigeria, Mozambique, Togo, Somalia, and Tanzania, among other African countries.

Copra, dried coconut endosperm, is an edible cooking oil that is also used cosmetically. Copra is called *mbata* by Swahili people and *igi agbon* by Yoruba. Whatever the name, it provides villages with milk for cooking and beverages, a base for molasses, and precious oil. Coconut oil–based soap forms a thick lather, even in saltwater, making it popular with seafaring people for thousands of years.

HARVESTING, COLLECTING AND USING COCONUT

When we lived on an island, one source of our daily food was coconut. The ripened ones fall from the tree, or they can be shaken from the branches, though sometimes it involves some tree climbing. When on the mainland and shopping for coconut, choose a coconut with a smooth, chestnut brown hull, with no apparent holes or mold. Shake and listen for a water sound. If it still contains water, it will be moist and tasty.

Bore two holes in the eyes using an ice pick or a sharp knife. The eyes are the dark brown spots at either end of the coconut. Pour the coconut water into a bowl. You can use this water for many purposes, adding it to your bath or pouring it over your head to condition your hair, or in other beauty recipes. Coconut water can also be used in rituals and ceremonies that honor appropriate orisha. Hit the hull on a hard surface sharply a few times—it should crack open. You can also hit the nut with a mallet or hammer. Once the coconut is cracked open, scoop out the flesh, which is called coconut meat, to use in recipes, or eat it as is.

HISTORY OF COCONUT IN THE DIASPORA

During early African American history, black people had many uses for the coconut. The shell was pulverized and consumed with wine as a systemic tonic. It was used to accelerate the movement of the blood and was deemed a favorable herb for the elders. Like the calabash, the coconut shell was made into numerous household tools such as cups, measuring containers, bowls, spoons, and small plates. In the Caribbean, coconut groves were where enslaved people went to commune with nature and relax.[18]

Making Coconut Milk

Heat 1½ cups water in a kettle, on medium-high heat. Meanwhile, grate the coconut flesh and put it in a sieve over a large bowl. Just before the water comes to a boil, pour it over the grated coconut in the sieve slowly. Press the coconut meat with the back of a wooden spoon. Discard the meat. Pour this liquid into a Pyrex measuring cup with a spout. Repeat this step three to four times. This makes about 1¼ cups rich coconut milk. (Tasty, tasty, tasty!)

Coconut Cream

To make coconut cream, bring 1½ cups whole milk almost to a boil. Go through the steps of making of coconut milk, using the milk instead of water. Coconut cream is a bit denser, with a full-bodied and sweeter taste, just right for desserts and drinks.

Toasted Coconut

Remove the coconut meat from the hull with sharp knife and shred. Add a tablespoon of olive oil to a cast iron skillet on medium heat. Add a pinch of sea salt, if desired. Add the shredded coconut meat and toss until it turns medium brown. Use this as a topping for fruit salads, yogurt, or cereal or eat alone, as a high-protein, low-carb snack.

Coconut oil can be a polarizing substance in the herbal community—some love it, while others despise it. It is said to be drying to the skin, particularly if used as a large part of a soap oil base, yet many African body butters are thick emollients that might overwhelm normal or combination skin, making coconut oil a welcomed lighter oil.

Coconut soaps are very useful for cleansing oily skin, as they make a frothy cleansing lather. For those who enjoy light moisturizer, coconut cream or other coconut products may well do the trick. Coconut oil can be combined with cocoa butter or shea butter to create a balanced soap, neither too astringent nor excessively emollient. Coconut cream is gaining popularity as a natural botanical for skin and hair care.

The skincare treatment gleaned from coconut is coconut cream, and not the type in the food aisle. Coconut cream is available from Togo, where women villagers hand-press coconuts to extract this creamy oil. This virgin coconut oil is pressed from fresh coconut milk and meat, rather than copra. Coconut cream works well as a massage therapy oil because of its silky texture.

In Africa, coconut cream has been used traditionally as a hair conditioner, strengthener, and growth aid. Coconut oil is rubbed into the scalp and may also be applied to the ends. The oil is melted, then cooled slightly and applied to the scalp and ends as a hot oil treatment, followed by a shampoo; this is preferable for those with oily scalps. I find that, when applying coconut cream to my face and hands, it is a butter that disappears within a minute or so, without leaving a trace of greasiness on the skin in the way that shea butter can.

Miraculous Acai: Brazilian Rainforest Magick

Euterpe oleracea Mart., commonly called acai (pronounced ah-SIGH-ee), is a palm tree growing in the rainforests of Brazil and elsewhere in South America. The skin of the palm tree's berry is the part that is garnering public attention as a superfood with miraculous healing qualities.

The excitement stems from the high amounts of age-defying antioxidants the berry's skin contains. The flavonoids it contains block diseased cells. A recent study shows that the bioactive polyphenolics present in acai berry reduce the proliferation of certain leukemia cells, in a dose and time-dependent manner.

In addition, acai berry skin is chock-full of amino acids and essential fatty acids. Acai is prepared and applied topically as shampoo, conditioner, leave-in conditioner, gel, balm, and pomade. Acai berry is a holistic healing herb that can be taken in capsule form and still benefit vitality. It can be enjoyed as a refreshing juice drink, or the pulp can be blended to make an energizing smoothie.

Unlike some distasteful health foods, the acai berry has a vibrant taste, similar to dark chocolate–covered cherries, or blueberry ice cream with chocolate flakes. Just this morning, I had some chilled acai juice, sweetened with a touch of agave, for a satisfying breakfast. It tastes very interesting, which entices us to enjoy it for its many other positive attributes, which include greater energy and vitality, increased stamina, better circulation, easier digestion, deeper sleep, and more satisfying sexual function.

Acai berry contains an array of vitamins, minerals, amino acids, and essential fatty acids. It has more protein per weight than eggs. Acai berry contains good concentrations of vitamins B2, B3, and E, and omega-3, -6, and -9 essential fatty acids. The fatty acid content is similar to that of olive oil. It is also rich in oleic acid, a monounsaturated antioxidant.

ESSENTIAL FATTY ACIDS

Omega-3
Alpha linolenic acid (ALA) is the primary omega-3 fatty acid. Omega-3s are helpful in forming cell walls, keeping them flexible, and improving circulation and oxygen intake. Omega-3s help with mental abilities and memory. Deficient omega-3s contribute to poor vision, blood clots, poor immunity, increased triglycerides, and bad cholesterol at increased levels. Deficiency in omega-3s also contributes to high blood pressure, irregular heartbeat, learning disorders, and slower growth in infants, children, and fetuses. It also contributes to menopausal discomfort.

Omega-6
The omega-6 contained in acai berry skin, called linoleic acid, lends numerous overall health benefits. Linoleic acid is the primary omega-6 fatty acid. Omega-6s can improve diabetic conditions, rheumatoid arthritis, PMS, and skin problems like eczema and psoriasis, and can help with cancer treatments. While many of us get an excess of linoleic acid in our diets, it is not converted into useful gamma linoleic acid (GLA) because of metabolic problems due to the consumption of sugar, alcohol, and trans fats from processed foods, along with smoking, pollution, stress, aging, viral infections, and other illnesses.

Omega-9
Oleic acid, called omega-9, is not considered an essential acid; however, it still contains significant health benefits. Omega-9 lowers the risk of heart attack and arteriosclerosis, and helps with cancer prevention.

ORAC stands for "oxygen radical absorbance capacity," a measurement of the antioxidants in foods. Healthy consumption of ORAC-rich foods helps prevent premature aging. Scientists believe that we need between 2,400 and 3,000 units of ORAC for their health benefits. A one-ounce serving of acai pulp juice, prepared from the berry skin, contains a whooping 3,800 units of ORAC.

Another important constituent of acai is anthocyanin. This constituent also provides some of the health benefit of red wine, yet the amount of anthocyanins in acai berry is ten to thirty-three times more, and twice as many as blueberries.

Acai Smoothie

I can live, and quite nicely, I might add, with an acai smoothie every morning, or, when cutting calories, simply the juice. The beverage combines juices such as guava, acai, banana, and apple.

I like to mix soft fruits with ice cubes in the blender to make a basic smoothie—this makes it smooth. Then, if I have energy left, I'll juice my own apples to add liquid to the smoothie as it is being blended, or use a prepared unsweetened, organic apple juice.

½ pouch of frozen acai puree (unsweetened preferable)

½ frozen banana

½ cup guava juice

½ cup unsweetened organic apple juice

1 teaspoon organic flaxseed

⅛ teaspoon finely ground cinnamon

⅛ teaspoon finely ground nutmeg

You can add a scoop of soy, whey, or rice and pea protein powder to boost the protein content. You can also add a tablespoon of unsweetened, unflavored yogurt and honey to taste. I find the addition of protein powder makes this a complete breakfast, and it tides me over until lunchtime.

Whatever you decide to use, add ingredients in the order given to the blender. Blend on medium until smooth. Add more apple juice if needed.

The combination of acai berry's vitamins, minerals, phytonutrients, EFAs, and chemical constituents come together to greatly benefit the hair and skin. While acai doesn't contain the full B complex, the B vitamins it does contain are known to strengthen hair, encouraging its growth. Having deficient B vitamins in the system contributes to dry scalp, greasy hair, dandruff, retarded hair growth, graying hair, wrinkled skin, parched lips, dry skin, irritations, and a red complexion. These vitamins could be taken orally, but many doctors are now recommending obtaining them through foods that contain them, such as acai.

Combined with the protein in acai, its vitamin C creates collagen. Collagen is essential for healthy skin. Ample C deters sagging skin and wrinkles. Vitamin C is responsible for keeping the skin moist, preventing lines and crinkling and stopping spider veins, tangled hair, and hair breakage by regulating the sebaceous glands. In addition, vitamin C benefits the eyes, teeth, the immune system, healing of wounds, and firming of skin tissue.

Vitamin E is known to help prevent wrinkles and the premature aging of skin and hair. The vitamin E in acai prevents dry, lifeless skin, hair breakage, and dandruff. It improves the healing of scars and wounds, as well as the circulation. Acai also contains calcium, which contributes to hair growth, strength, and healthy condition; phosporus; potassium, which regulates circulation; and protein. Hair is primarily made of the protein keratin. Diets deficient in protein lead to all sorts of hair problems, including hair breakage, slow hair growth, and thinning. Adequate amounts of protein in the diet are believed to accentuate hair growth, strength, and condition. Acai also contains a healthy amount of amino acids, which are constantly required by the hair follicles to maintain hair growth.

Honoring the Quebradeiras de Coco: The Story of Babassu

Like many of the wildcrafted organic butters and oils I've written about, babassu is intimately tied to women, fair trade, tradition, and community. Unlike shea butter, however, babassu has not yet become a household name.

Babassu palms (*Orbignya phalerata*) grow along the southern and northeastern edge of the Brazilian Amazon. Ironically, it flourishes in economically challenged provinces such as Maranhao. The babassu palm also grows in parts of Mexico and Guyana. The trees grow up to sixty feet tall, and occupy almost twenty-nine million hectares of forest. In its native areas, it forms the dominant plant coverage. Because of the health and prosperity it lends, it is considered by many to be a Tree of Life.

Babassu has over thirty-five uses, ranging from attracting game to acting as an insect repellent. Though it may sound foreign to many, in the Amazon of Brazil babassu palm is thoroughly utilized and recognized as a very sustainable plant. Most of its usefulness is derived from the seed kernels within the fruits. The fruit resembles small coconuts and grows in bunches ranging from a few dozen to hundreds. The mature fruit falls from the tree, mainly from August to November, but this continues into January and February, which is the time the rainy season begins.

The seeds contain an oil that is in the spotlight for hair care. It is added to shampoos, conditioners, and pomades. The seed kernels are cold pressed to produce the oil, and the fruits are wildcrafted and organic. Cold pressing means pressure is used to extract the oil, rather than chemical solvents, making this a very wholesome oil.

Indigenous and other people use babassu oil (where it grows as a native plant) as a moisturizer. The oil is noted for its light feel and the fact that it is easily absorbed into the skin. It is preferred over heavier oils because of its nongreasy application. Surprisingly, it works as well for oily skin as it does for dry skin because it is an adaptable oil.

The leaves of babassu palm are used to create thatch-roof housing, woven mats, and walls. The stems are strong and woody, lending themselves to usefulness as timbers.

The oil is very high in essential fatty acids, making it ideal for many purposes. Babassu oil is also high in lauric acid. Lauric acid is very low in toxicity, lending to its use in body care. Lauric acid is solid at room temperature, melting from touch. Babassu oil also contains high concentrations of myristic acid. Lauric and myristic acids draw body heat, lending babassu oil what herbalists call coolant and refrigerant qualities—it cools down the skin and scalp, making it useful in the summer, after sunburn, and when blow drying or using heat on the hair. Babassu contains a significant amount of oleic acid, which lends to its healthful quality when consumed. Oils with good concentrations of oleic acid are known to lower blood cholesterol. Like most palms, babassu contains palmitic acid. Palmitate, an antioxidant, and vitamin A compound are also found in babassu.

Babassu forms a protective, soothing coating on skin or hair. It is helpful in the effort to withstand diverse weather conditions and protect against direct-heat styling tools, while also limiting the damage from color treatments or other chemicals. It leaves the skin feeling velvety and supple. Babassu has superior emollient qualities—emollients draw moisture from the air, lending skin, nails, or hair a healthful glow.

Multipurpose babassu is also used for cooking and to make cosmetics such as creams, soaps, shower gels, powders, and body butters. Other products made with the seed oil include animal feed, beverages, flour, and healing remedies.

Next are featured indigenous women (not descended from Africa) whose work embodies the confluence of sustainability, ritual, folklore, and holistic health so central to utilizing African tree medicine for the New World.

FAIR TRADE AND QUEBRADEIRAS DE COCO (NUT BREAKERS)

In the late 1970s, indigenous people utilized the babassu palm as a way of defining community—the trees were used to make a stand against loggers and cattle farmers, who were clear-cutting babassu-rich Amazon forests. *Quebradeiras de Coco* are primarily women. The women chanted and performed rituals in the forest to warn loggers and farmers off their trees. Eventually they met with success. The indigenous people who have revered these trees for over four hundred years occupy the Maranhao region of Brazil and continue to incorporate the babassu into their lives.

Today, commercial activity around babassu palm affects the income of over two million rural Brazilians. Babassu is even used as local currency in some areas. People are allowed to exchange nuts for goods and services once a week. Women continue to sing, chant, and perform rituals around the harvesting and processing of babassu nuts.

Women gather and collect the ripened fruit from atop the earth, placing them in handwoven baskets. Fruits are gathered; the inner nut is extremely tough, but women crack it open using wooden clubs, sweat, and perseverance. Inside the nut is an oil-rich kernel, the outer hull of which is used for charcoal and burned during oil processing, lending sustainability even to its industrial extraction. Babassu oil sales to cosmetics firms are regulated by fair trade organizations. The money generated from its sale helps otherwise severely impoverished areas and families gain a viable income. In short, buying any type of wholesome products featuring babassu helps improve the lifestyle and living conditions of many people living in Brazil.

Murumuru

Murumuru and *murui* are the Portuguese names for *Astrocaryum murumuru*. In Spanish, this tree is called *chonta*, *chuchana*, and *huicongo*. Murumuru is in the family *arecaceae*, the genus *Astrocaryum*, and the species *Murumuru*. The plant has spines or sharp edges, requiring proper precaution during harvest. Murumuru is prickled everywhere, even the seeds and flowers.

Murumuru grows in the Amazon basins, enjoying a distinctive place in local ecosystems as one of the dominant trees. It grows particularly well in northern Brazil, especially Maranhao. Finding the tree on your own could prove tricky, however, because the species varies radically. It can be short and without stems, or tall, with more than one robust trunk. Murumuru has a shuttlecock-like crown at the top, with large, flat leaves that have very closely spaced leaflets and silvery undersides. The large fruits are edible.

Oil is a common constituent of most types of seeds, and palms have large, abundant seeds. The murumuru palm nut is wildcrafted, meaning it is not cultivated. Many people prefer wildcrafted botanicals because they have not been treated with pesticides or fertilizers and are a very integrated part of their environment. Local people cherish murumuru nuts for their numerous contributions to health and wellness. They also hold a special place in the folklore and mythology of several areas.

The oil derived from murumuru nuts is used for many purposes. The large fruits are edible, and the seed kernel is a significant source of edible oil. The kernel also produces a rich extract used by the beauty industry for shampoos, conditioners, and skin care products. A rich lather is derived from its kernels, useful in soaps and shampoos.

Still, with so many types of oils available internationally, you might wonder why folks go through all the stinging prickles to get to the fruit and seed of murumuru in particular. For one, the lipids present in the plant material hydrate and moisturize skin and hair intensively. The emolliency supports the integrity of your skin and your hair's cutaneous barrier. Moreover, murumuru is chock-full of nurturing vitamins and minerals that are generally beneficial to the body. The nutty aroma of organic murumuru puts us in touch with Mother Earth, and it is a tangible part of the great Amazon rainforest.

Murumuru is especially useful to people of all ethnicities with kinky, curly, or wavy hair because of its softening ability. Frequently, kinky and some types of curly hair feel coarse. Murumuru coats coarse curls, making them more supple and manageable. Products containing an appreciative amount of murumuru oil or extract are well suited to textured curls. Murumuru products moisturize the hair with lasting hydration, control frizz, and define curls.

From the moment of their first meeting, Native American and African people shared with one another a respect for the life-giving forces of nature, of the earth. African settlers in Florida taught the Creek Nation run-aways, the "Seminoles," methods for rice cultivation. Native peoples taught recently arrived black folks all about the many uses of corn. . . . Sharing the reverence for the earth, black and red people helped one another remember that, despite the white man's ways, the land belonged to everyone.

—bell hooks, Sisters of the Yam[19]

The rich butter made from murumuru is a light amber color, with an earthen aroma. It is rich in oleic acid, which promotes overall good health. Oleic acid–rich botanicals aid with moisture retention, benefiting skin and hair. The emollient constituents in murumuru enhance the natural gloss of hair and provide sheen to naturally dull, kinky, or highly textured hair.

Murumuru ingredients also provide a healthy shine to chemically treated, overprocessed, or otherwise damaged hair. Murumuru, like babassu, is an economical botanical tree, and when wildcrafted and organic it provides much-needed income to the communities where it grows. It is used increasingly in sustainability projects and fair trade.

Saw Palmetto

Saw palmetto (*Serenoa repens*), called palm cabbage (Gullah), grows in areas where Gullah people lived for several hundred years in the Carolina lowlands. Gullah people have a tradition of using saw palmetto in their sweetgrass basketry, and this tradition continues today. There is a history, as well, of creating a palm wine called *maluvu* from the sap, juice, or center of the top of saw palmetto, the part the people call palm cabbage. Secret doctors and treaters of Louisiana use saw palmetto, which grows there equally well, in their healer's repertoire. In fact, this southern U.S. tree grows in Alabama and south throughout Florida. It grows abundantly in Florida as an understory plant of the forest, and provides beach growth. Saw palmetto grows along the Caribbean coastline and has some uses as a beverage there as well. It is commercially harvested from the wild in quite a dangerous production, because it is a prickly plant, protective of its precious berries.

Seminoles, who have a concentration of African ancestry, recognized saw palmetto fruits as a food, though they are tart, and used them as medicine as well. Seminoles prepare infusions of saw palmetto berries to treat upset stomach and diarrhea, and as a diuretic and sexual stimulant. The Lumbee, who identify as Native American but have some African ancestry as well, mainly of Robeson County, North Carolina, have a long history of using saw palmetto medicinally.*

---

*Intercultural mixing occurred when enslaved people escaped their owners and were taken in by the Seminole community. The Seminole are one of the more prominent groups of "Black Indians," an admixture of Native American and African American people.

Beneath many a saw palmetto tree is a discreetly situated eastern diamondback rattlesnake. Many symbols and omens are represented by the rattlesnake in snake mysticism. Snakes remain intricately tied to our tree medicine and healing ways in Africa and the New World. Whether this particular snake is a totem, omen, or protector of the tree remains to be considered. What we do know is that each year people are bitten when they do not realize that saw palmetto is the diamondback rattlesnake's hideout. Awareness and respect are key to the productive gathering and processing of tree medicines.

SAW PALMETTO AND BPH

Benign prostratic hypertrophy (BPH) diminishes quality of life for men, and over 50 percent of men over fifty experience it. Saw palmetto provides relief for many people with this condition. The most studied phyto-tree medicines for the prostate are extracts of saw palmetto fruit. In addition, saw palmetto fruit is associated with improving the libido in both sexes and reducing impotence in men.[20]

This chapter is a tribute to palms, one of the African diaspora's most significant trees. Palms hail from the forest, rainforest canopy (overstory), and understory. By yielding oils, berries, and nuts rich in antioxidants, essential oils, amino acids, and other phytonutrients, palms have an impressive role in complementary health. Moreover, these are trees that have a welcomed place in ancient African folklore and mythology while also serving an important role in divination and spirituality. As a true Tree of Life, with over twenty-six hundred species, palms provide rich healing motifs in all manners of our lives.

As you have seen throughout this chapter, palm oil is used in cosmetics, confections, baked goods, and for cooking. Babassu palm steps into a different arena. It has been utilized by indigenous people in a political manner, melding social justice, tradition, mythology, and sustainability. Within your home, not only will you have many palm products in the pantry and medicine cabinet, but inevitably you will also find palm tree parts serving utilitarian and decorative functions, in the form of cork (shoes, wine, bulletin boards, furniture), rattan (indoor and outdoor furniture and basketry), fronds as woven goods, nuts carved and used as jewelry and buttons, and even a sustainable and "green" furniture wax.

The role of palms traverses the mundane into the spiritual dimension with ease. Palm trees are sites of petitions and offerings to deity, the ancestors, and nature spirits. Parts

---

Saw Palmetto Tea

The ratio of this tea is 1 teaspoon of dried saw palmetto berries to 1 cup of water. Decoct for 20 minutes. Strain, sweeten if desired, and drink.

of the tree are employed in divination because of the palm's social and metaphysical stature in the black and brown communities. Keeping the traditional community safe from negative energy, palms are even used in seasonal rituals—their purpose to arbitrate between humans and the wild spirits of the sacred wood. These are some of the reasons I have devoted this, the final chapter, to palm trees.

EPILOGUE

Seeds of Hope

PARTICIPATION IN VILLAGES FAR AND WIDE

Environmentalism, sustainability, and agroforestry projects have been given a white face in the media, which shapes the hearts and minds of many Americans. No doubt, they have been white-washed. In fact, in a recent article by Cliff Hocker in *Black Enterprise*, when African Americans are asked about their concern over pollution of the air and water or exposure to toxic substances, they consistently report more concern than whites for community blight and environmental hazards.[1] This goes for Latino communities as well, according to a 2003 study by University of Michigan Professor Paul Mohai, "Dispelling Old Myths: African American Concern for the Environment."

Another study done by Mohai and associates in Detroit in 2002 discredited the belief that blacks only cared about their own neighborhoods—their concern for the global environment far exceeded that of whites. These studies also showed a marked participation in environmental activism on the part of African Americans. Blacks outdid whites in pro-environmental lifestyle choices, in terms of buying organic food, driving less (taking public transportation and carpooling), and eating less meat. According to Hocker, "what appears as low African American engagement with sustainability and environmentalism is an illusion."[2] The difference that may lead to lower recording of our participation is that African Americans often form their own community groups. Black participation in the green movement began to pick up steam in the 1980s, and at the time it was referred to as "environmental justice."

The interesting thing about whitewash is that it is just a skim coat of paint over a more complex structure. Once we peel back the layers—and not too far back, mind you—we find that indigenous and African-descended people are as committed as any other groups to these causes. This epilogue investigates agroforestry, fair trade, and micro-industry projects in Africa's diaspora, in villages near and far. Seeds of Hope are black people on the front lines trying to forge change in their environment.

The Cautionary Tale of Mapou, Haiti

So far in this book we have had a wonderful journey through the conceptual African forest. I have shared some of my personal forest stories, how they began as almost a source of shame and instead became central in my creativity and my healing lifestyle. I have described how my kinship to trees developed and where I am with it now in the hope that it might inspire those without such a relationship to cultivate one. Mostly I have spoken positively of a wonderful living history shared by people of African descent with trees, but there is always a downside; this is the duality of life. I want to share the cautionary tale of *mapou* so that the importance of trees to the ecosystem and to people of all colors is etched firmly in the psyche.

Silk cottonwood (*Ceiba pentandra*), majestic native of West Africa, the Caribbean, and North and South America, is one tree that immediately comes to mind as an example of the importance of sustainability to black communities. The people of Haiti call the silk cottonwood *mapou*. Like many of the trees discussed in these pages, *mapou* is considered sacred. It was once illegal to fell the trees, one way indigenous people have protected their natural resources. This tree had religious significance; offerings were laid out at the base, within the buttresses, nooks, and crannies of *mapou*, just as they are with the Angel Oak and other silk cotton trees throughout Africa and the diaspora. As a sacred tree, *mapou* is believed to be the container of the ancestors. The roots are said to contain the vodou lwas and spirits. When a child is born, the father buries the umbilical cord of the baby at *mapou*. The tree holds the baby's soul and, as we know, children are the future generations of societies to come. This brings us back to the notion of the sacred union of spirit and living beings by the silk cottonwood tree.

Taino people, who are indigenous to Haiti, named the tree *mapu*, meaning large red tree. We have learned of the spiritual significance of red in African cultures on both sides of the Atlantic. *Mapou* grows to an enormous size in places where most trees remain saplings. The trunk is hollow, with numerous branches and cavities. It requires a reliable water source. It does not supply a good source of lumber, and was traditionally valued for shade, spiritual engagement, folklore, mythology, and spirit medicine.

Eventually, it was discovered that it makes a good source for charcoal. Charcoal was sold for pennies per pound, bringing income, however tiny, to very impoverished people. Today, the place named for the great tree, Mapou, Haiti, does not have a single *mapou* left. A period of massive deforestation severely disrupted the ecosystem and holistic environment in Haiti. The primary beliefs of the people, and their homage to their ancestral spirits, were severed along with the trees. Whether one believes in tree spirits or not, the fact remains that an estimated twenty-five hundred people were killed by a great flood in June 2004. Approximately sixteen hundred victims came from Mapou and its environs. The trees serve the spirit; they offer medicine and an opportunity to commune with the ancestors. As the cautionary tale of Mapou, Haiti, shows, trees also have a very important ecological function. Their roots soak up water, and forests form barriers, stemming the tide of erosion. In short, trees play an important role in balancing our ecosystem and sustaining life.

> Mapou mouri, kabrit manje fey.
> *When the mapou dies, goats would eat its leaves.*

This Haitian proverb attests to the role that *mapou* played in the life cycles of the community. *Mapou* had a very important place in the cycle of life, continuity, and balance in Haiti; unfortunately, a notion of a different type of survival, based on economics, disrupted this.

We fight to regain our natural legacy by land and by sea.

Starving for What We Had

In Swahili, *Harambee* means "Let's all pull together."[3] This is the motto for the Green Belt Movement. *Harambee*, through the Green Belt Movement, or GBM, sees trees, land, community, and survival as being inextricable. A remarkable woman named Wangari Maathai started this movement.

One of the first public acts by GBM was a tree ceremony. Wangari felt her people were forgetting the importance of their elders and ancestors. The first tree ceremony organized by her group in 1977 honored recently deceased Kenyan ancestors. For her, ancestors and living people bring abundance and prosperity to the community, through knowledge and positive spirit. Trees were planted to honor the ancestors. This was followed by a national campaign aimed at informing the public of the dangers of desertification, and actions necessary to reverse destruction.

As we saw with *mapou* in Haiti, one of the ironies of Westernization is that, with its implied improvements on more "primitive" conditions, sometimes just the opposite occurs. In Kenya, for example, environment and community were very negatively impacted once outsiders took an interest in the country's land. Sustainable, economically viable, nutritious traditional crops such as banana, papaya, acacia, and avocado were replaced by land- and water-hungry cash crops like sugar cane and coffee. As seemingly convenient foods, processed and packaged, replaced indigenous foods, families found they had to strain to find money to pay for such luxuries, and needed appropriate ways to prepare these foreign foods using traditional means—typically an open wood fire. Many went hungry. The community was slowly becoming as eroded and depleted as the land. Outsiders grew rich from Kenyan land while the native people and their environment became impoverished.

Wangari Maathai's way of changing the world, bringing stability and holistic health to her country and improving the situation of Africans and rural women in particular, is her passion for nature and tradition. She started GBM as a grassroots, feminist-based NGO (non-governmental organization) focused on environmental conservation and development. She began a grassroots tree-planting campaign as the core activity of the group. Members are from mostly rural areas, and are primarily women.[4] Maathai's GBM goals are to:

>> **Fight malnutrition through environmental conservation.** Implement programs to fight malnutrition, widespread poverty, unemployment, underemployment, overpopulation, energy crises, soil erosion, lack of clean drinking water, building materials, animal fodder, drought, and desertification.[5] Steer people away from packaged, processed, or canned foods, which are not wholesome and are difficult to cook on the wood stoves many people use, and are also too expensive to buy in enough quantity to sustain poor rural families, thus leading to malnutrition. GBM urges people to return to eating more traditional foods like indigenous fruits and wildcrafted foods. Legumes like black beans, butter beans, and pigeon peas are sustainable and affordable nutritious foods that are promoted, along with maize, millet, and sorghum. The hallmark is the banana tree, which traditionally grew in the rich stands of forest in the area. The driving force behind GBM is to know one's botanical and cultural roots.

» **Stem the threat of the complete deforestation of Kenya** by planting stands of trees and indigenous grasses to stop soil erosion, exploring substitutes for the wood fuel and trees used as fodder, and implementing ways to plan construction and infrastructure. This goal was met through community education initiatives.

» **Empower people at the grassroots** through a variety of schemes built around sustainable farming, forestry, and agroforestry.

» **Help people establish sustainable fuel sources.** Over 90 percent of rural people are poor and depend on inexpensive, readily available forms of fuel such as grain stalks, wood, and cow dung. Women, who are farmers and gatherers, began to have to work harder, extending their range for gathering, and then carrying lumber back to their homes for use as fuel.

» **Rectify troubling issues in farming.** Traditionally, women were responsible for cultivating annual crops, which were stored in granaries, while men were in charge of perennial crops. With the rise in colonization, this social structure was disrupted; gradually, farming became almost exclusively the domain of women, who are already overstretched by other societal obligations. Over the years, many farmers ignored organic and other sustainable methods of farming, convinced that chemical fertilizers were better. GBM promotes organic farming, the use of animal manure, mulching, composting, sustainable farming methods, and community education about food production and nutrition. Crop rotation was also instilled by GBM, to add nutrients to the soil and minimize the net change in soil.[6]

» **Harvesting water.** GBM uses damming, benching, mulching, pitting, cut-off drains, terracing, manure application, double digging, contour farming, furrowing, and agroforestry; all of these are techniques that conserve and trap water and slow the rate of water run-off.[7]

» **Train women who are underemployed or unemployed** by building skills in nutrition, traditional food preparation, farming, natural product manufacture, and establishing and maintaining nurseries, forestry, and agroforestry.

» **Instill traditional values.** One of the important hallmarks of GBM is instilling environmental consciousness and traditional values among youth, including respect for nature, the importance of traditional foods, and the holistic health of community vital to the people before colonization. The restoration of positive spiritual and cultural values is seen as an important way to build self-confidence, empowering identity, which in turns protects indigenous biological diversity, earth-based wisdom, and practical knowledge.[8]

AFRICA'S MOST PROMINENT ENVIRONMENTALIST AND NOBEL PRIZE WINNER

While we've become familiar with African men like Desmond Tutu (spiritual leader), Nelson Mandela (civil rights activist), and Kofi Annan (former secretary general of the United Nations) bringing attention to issues of importance to international cooperation and world peace, today a group of women are coming to the fore. The Green Belt Movement is the brainchild of Wangari Maathai, a Kikuya woman from the Nyeri district of central Kenya at the foot of Mt. Kenya. GBM's way of changing the world, bringing stability and holistic health and improving the situation of Africans and rural women in particular, is through their passion for nature and tradition.

Over twenty years ago, Wangari Maathai started GBM with a grassroots tree-planting campaign as the core activity of the group. Members are mostly from rural areas, and are primarily women.[9] Dr. Maathai holds a Ph.D. in veterinarian medicine. She accepted a position as a visiting fellow at Yale University's Global Institute for Sustainable Forestry in 2002. Maathai was appointed to Kenya's Parliament in 2003. She is an Elder of the Burning Spear, and the first sub-Saharan African woman to win a Nobel Peace Prize. Maathai won the Nobel Peace Prize for her work in ecologically sustainable development. She has been applauded for working for peace using a holistic approach, encompassing democracy, environmentalism, human rights, and women's rights. Her work through GBM combines sciences, social commitment, and political activism.

The Movement

In her book *The Green Belt Movement: Sharing the Approach and the Experience*, Maathai states that the cause of malnutrition, deforestation, and impending desertification was that people were disrupted from their traditional ways of life by colonialism. Contemporary Kenyans seemed to prefer a Western lifestyle to their own traditions, even though they did not have the means, sacrificing what riches they had.

Today, Maathai's group is beloved by environmentalists around the world. It has planted over thirty million trees to prevent soil erosion, provide firewood for cooking fires, and increase the health and welfare of her people. Her organization maintains a nine-acre education center. Not content to stay within Kenya, a Pan-African Green Belt Network was established in 1986, with broad-based tree-planting programs in several other African nations, including Tanzania, Uganda, Malawi, Lesotho, Ethiopia, and Zimbabwe. All together, millions have been educated about the connection between a healthy environment and sustainable development because of GBM. In the Resources and Organizations section, you will see how you can join this important organization and become involved in its work.

Founded in the United States in 1975, Students in Free Enterprise (SIFE) is a global not-for-profit education organization dedicated to improving quality of life and standard of living. SIFE is about teaching people of various education levels the principles and values of free-market economics. Working in partnership with businesses and higher education and using natural resources and indigenous knowledge, SIFE organizes, trains, and motivates teams of university students to teach others within the community an understanding of free enterprise.

A Successful Soapmaking Initiative at the University of Ghana

I have been fortunate to make yet another new friend in Africa, Johann, a native of Ghana and fellow soapmaker. He has been sharing the progress of a soapmaking project with me through e-mail. The project was aimed at Kpomkpo, a farming village in the greater Accra region. According to the sponsoring organization, the people live in abject poverty despite the fact that they engage in seasonal farming and have large tracts of cultivable land available. They have an abundance of palm fruits, an essential ingredient in soap production. With strategic planning, the people set out to make a profitable palm soap industry to serve as an income-generating venture using their natural resources.

The objective for the project was to tap into the resources of these people to help reduce area poverty. A group of people were selected and trained in the production of soap for their immediate market and subsequently for other areas. Since most of the people are illiterate, contacting potential participants was done in person. No fee was charged to participate, and certificates of completion were given at the end of the program. Resource persons held practical sessions to train fifteen to twenty participants at a time. The training involved practical soapmaking, basic bookkeeping, and marketing. The project lasted one semester. The target market was the local people of Kpomkpo and the surrounding communities and villages. Eventually it was intended to extend out to include the main markets of Accra, depending on the creation of high-quality soap. The group's philosophy is: "We are what we repeatedly do. Excellence, then, is not an act but a habit."

Corporate and Community: Meeting Through Botanicals

Elsewhere, companies buy raw botanicals gathered and prepared for use by indigenous people. For example, Aveda and The Body Shop buy their oils directly from indigenous women's collectives such as the Cooperative of Agro-Extractivist Producers (COPALJ). The two companies have done a great deal to bring babassu and those who harvest and process it to the attention of the international community, seeking fair treatment. COPALJ consists of a dozen communities in the Maranhao area. The collective collects the nuts, presses the nuts into oil, and sells the product to the international marketplace.

AGROFORESTRY

When agroforestry makes economic and social sense, by meshing with traditions, it greatly improves the holistic health of the community. This is being clearly illustrated by the work of SIFE, GBM, and COPALJ. Successful agroforestry embraces the sustainable uses of trees, supports the spiritual, religious, and cultural significance of trees within their communities, and supports the development of NTFPs like soap and other utilitarian and decorative crafts. Some of these programs include frankincense, myrrh, and acacia, used in incense; tree medicines for healing; trees for consumption in a wildcrafted indigenous diet rich in fruit, nuts, arils, kernels, and other tree parts that provide sustenance and economic returns; sensitive harvesting of the medicinal parts of plants; the use of plant fibers in papermaking and other schemes; and sustaining the wildlife associated with the trees. Agroforestry may consist of informal plantations, such as locales where shea trees are tended, community woodlots, and communally owned and operated plantations. Sacred groves are an ancient way that forests have sustained holistic health.

TAMMIE UMBEL OF TERRA SHEA

Recently I had the opportunity to try a lovely shea butter with a golden color, imported by the African Shea Butter Company. I enjoy the golden shea butter immensely, because it retains the smells of the open wood fires on which it was created. This is likely to be a sentiment shared by those who work with herbs, because it reminds us of the power of the elements.

Delving into a jar of golden shea butter can spiritually transport the user back to the African village in which it was processed. Those of you who seek a more unprocessed product, with a lively spirit still intact, would be wise to avoid ultrarefined shea butter, which is stripped of its contact with its source.

African Shea Butter/Terra Shea is a woman-owned and -operated mail-order firm. I had the pleasure of interviewing Tammie Umbel, the founder and sole proprietor of this company, while she was pregnant with her tenth child. During our conversation, it was apparent that the African Shea Butter Company's main objective is helping African people through trade and the use of traditional methods, materials, and indigenous plants.

Umbel contracts with African soapmakers and wraps her soap line in traditionally dyed African fabric and indigenous papers. African Shea Butter Company sells a variety of high-grade shea butters in bulk, suitable for use by the most discerning herbalist. Umbel is reaching out to other African women's harvesting and manufacturing cooperatives; she now carries baobab, argan, and black seed oil as well as African-grown and -processed lemongrass and bourbon geranium essential oils. The support of UNIFEM, L'Occitane, African Shea Butter Company, and numerous other governmental organizations and NGOs is enabling women's groups to pool their resources and purchase simple presses, which lessen their physical labor. West African women are receiving technical training from organizations such as SIFE and learning to create and market their own natural cosmetics and healing balms.

We've Known Permaculture for a Very Long Time

"The Forest is our home; when we leave the forest, or when the forest dies, we shall die. We are the people of the forest."[10]
> —Old Moke, a BaMbuti pymy of the Ituri Forest, Congo,
> central Africa, recorded in the early 1960s

The indigenous people around the world are often spoken of in the past tense. It is as though they are all gone and their way of life is only a part of our collective past. There is nothing further from the truth—there are significant numbers of indigenous people living in Africa and the Americas. Nevertheless, locked into this mind-set that is based more on an agreed-upon mythology than fact, people look to Westernized societies for lessons of how to live in harmony with nature. Two Canadian men, Dr. Bill Mollison and David Holmgren, coined the word *permaculture* in the early 1970s. It is a descriptor for a sustainable way of life.

Permaculture, or *permanent agriculture*, as it is known today, is the conscious design and maintenance of agriculturally productive ecosystems that are diverse, stable, and resilient. It is also a way of bringing together landscape and people, creating a symbiotic relationship. Environmental harmony is created when people, animals, and the environment have their holistic needs met through permanent agriculture. This circular relationship in turn becomes sustainable.

When I wanted to learn from a culture that has practiced permaculture for thousands of years, I did not look to North America; instead, I headed off to Australia for an extended study with various Aboriginal cultures. The Aborigines are numerous, diverse groups who live in vastly different ecosystems. They have managed their land

and ecosystems respectfully, in accord with steeped tradition, for over fifty thousand years. While some live in tropical coastal environs, many people have managed over the generation in harsh desert environments.

Increasingly, other people from various walks of life are paying attention to environmental programs modeled after the traditional ways of life of the indigenous cultures. As you shall see in the following examples, there are lessons for how to live a healthful life being developed and disseminated from the Motherland to this very day.

The Man Who Stands by the Mangrove with Spirit

Sometimes, one person feeling the power of a natural environment can spark a movement. Such is the case with a lone voice in the woods, Wadja Egnankou, a scientist from the Ivory Coast. Egnankou fought long and hard to bring attention to the irreplaceable nature of his nation's mangroves. The Ivorian mangroves are an incredibly diverse biome, providing space for interchange between the Atlantic Ocean and tropical rainforest. The mangroves are densely populated with microorganisms and act as a nursery for fish and shellfish, which are key food sources for many coastal people.

"The mangrove forests are a terrestrial paradise. I will do whatever is necessary to save them."[11]
—*Wadja Egnankou*

In 1992, Egnankou was awarded the prestigious Goldman Environmental Prize for his work raising grassroots awareness concerning the treasures of the mangrove. The destruction of mangrove forests would have catastrophic results on the environment, society, and local economies. His work included hiring a team of experts to show the local government how to build roads outside the mangrove areas, thereby keeping the ecosystem intact. It brought him and his cause international attention.

Without one person standing up against their destruction in his country, the mangroves would likely have been quietly destroyed. A long-term professor at the University of Abidjan, Egnankou has been on leave, working to implement a Global Environmental Facility to curb a new threat, the invasion of exotic vegetation.

American Grassroots Activists

We have many examples of grassroots activists in the United States as well. One is a seemingly ordinary woman who stood up to the mysterious powers of the corporate world to clean her town of dis-ease and despair. Margie Eugene-Richard had long suspected that the Shell Oil chemical plant and refinery that bordered her Norco, Louisiana, neighborhood was contributing to the respiratory illnesses and other ailments that plagued her family and neighbors. Margie's neighborhood was actually called Cancer Alley by local people. It is a historically African American community called Old Diamond. The house she grew up in was just twenty-five feet away from the plant's fence line.

Now sixty-two, Richard fought the hard fight to sweep clean her neighborhood, leading a battle on the front lines to hold Shell accountable for the devastating health problems in her neighborhood. Four generations of Richard's family lived in Old Diamond, which is near the southern Mississippi River. Many of its residents reported high rates of cancer, birth defects, and other serious health ailments. Most of the neighbors, like Richard's family, lived within four square blocks sandwiched between the Shell plant and a Motiva oil refinery. Over a third of the children in the town suffered from asthma or bronchitis. Richard's sister died at age forty-three from sarcoidosis, a rare bacterial infection. The Shell plant has been a fixture in Norco, which is twenty-five miles west of New Orleans, since 1920. It has looming tanks and belching vapor stacks that could fill nine football fields. The corporation has been buying out local residents, most of whom are descendants of enslaved people or sharecroppers, to expand.

The event that motivated Richard, who was then a middle school teacher, to take action using legal channels was a blast in 1973 from a Shell pipeline that knocked a house off its foundation, killing an elder and a teenage boy who was mowing the lawn. Another major accident occurred in 1988, when 159 million pounds of toxins were spewed into the air. Seven workers were killed. Richard began to mobilize her neighbors and family, the media, and environmentalists. In 2000, Shell agreed to reduce its emissions by 20 percent and improve emergency evacuation procedures for the town. Shell also voluntarily relocated residents who lived on the four streets closest to the plant, paying market value for the properties. Margie Eugene-Richard is the first African American to win the prestigious Goldman Environmental Prize.

Community Activism and Hands-On Healing

I have had the pleasure of meeting and working with herbalist Leah Paterson in my workshops. We now converse through my Yahoo study group. She is part of our younger generation of African American healers working holistically in the community. When I met Leah, she was working at a grassroots level as director of adult education at Garfield Conservatory, one of Chicago's finest plant research centers. Today, Paterson teaches health and beauty classes using minerals for personal care, and runs her own holistic cleaning company in North Carolina. She continues to create and sell her own herbal body care products as well. With an international vision, she hopes that some day all the facets of her work will come together to yield a positive impact internationally. Following is a statement from Paterson in response to my interview questions about her role in the community working with complementary medicine.

I began a nonprofit organization, Soulistic Sanctuary, to educate the minority community on holistic health and sustainable living practices. I'm currently pursuing my esthetics license to work more deeply with skin and hair care, two major areas of concern for most people. I plan to open an herbal wellness spa in the future. I became interested in holistic health as a research fellow at the National Institutes of Health. Seeing how patients often succumbed to their treatment over their disease impressed upon me that there must be a better way. That led me into holistic health. Realizing how much I had not learned about true health led me to learn and then bring the information to others, especially those who would not have normally come across it. I hope that my work will empower people to regain a solid connection with the earth, their innate intuition, and their inner selves. Practically, I want everyone to have the ability to walk outside his or her door and harvest something for whatever ails them. That encompasses many changes for the world today and that is the work I hope to help accomplish. I envision the black community regaining an innate healing wisdom in such a way that the knowledge and practice of holistic health becomes "commonplace." My work is helping our country realign itself with the wisdom of the rest of the world.

Rumor has it that Paterson is not only a fascinating herbalist and community health activist, but she is also thought of as one of the Chicago area's best dancers on the Latin scene. In this book, I have stressed the importance of including the arts to supplement health, wholeness, and well-being. I was curious about why Leah, who does so many things, also dances. I wondered if it might have a spiritual connection to her work. Leah responded, "My dancing began as an expression of the most intangible of my emotions and has grown to become an expression of my divinity and my full goddess nature as well. It has helped me to continue to blossom fully into what I think is true womanhood."

Natural Hair Care

One of the main tributaries bringing African Americans into the concept of "natural" is natural hair care. Where once we burned our hair and scalp and scorched the environment with chemicals, sizzling petroleum-based oils, and straightening tools, today people are increasingly reaching out to natural means. These means draw heavily on African tree medicines—natural soaps and shampoos, for example, are rich in coconut and palm. Shea butter is used in style products and for deep conditioning, as are the banana tree, avocado, mango, babassu, acai, murumuru, and many others discussed in these pages.

The burgeoning natural hair care industry gives entrepreneurs from Africa a way of sustaining themselves, providing a decent income. Most "braider" shops in cities like Chicago, for example, are owned and operated by women braiders from places like Côte D'Ivoire, Mali, Guinea, Burkino Faso, and Nigeria. These spaces allow intimate cultural interchanges between Africans and African Americans who may not have had previous contact with continental Africans. This in itself is a healing activity, making steps toward healing the deeply entrenched wounds African Americans have from being separated from the Motherland and sold into slavery.

For many years I frequented braider shops, wearing my hair in cornrows, extended microbraids, Senegalese twists, and Nubian knots. I transitioned my hair this way from a short 'fro, cut off to remove all traces of chemicals, to double-strand twists, which led to locs. I made friends with Yoruba through two women: Sharefa, a Nigerian muslim, and Nnedi, a popular author, both very different people yet both from Yorubaland.

I gained confidence in my African heritage and the beauty it could lend just from being around African women from various countries. This is one of the gifts of living in a cosmopolitan city like Chicago. Frequenting a preeminent braider's paradise like Amazon's Natural Look Salon, now located both on the south side of Chicago and Maui, Hawaii, as well as "hole in the wall" local braider's shops, I gained the opportunity to hear impromptu chants and songs as the women work and banter in local languages blended with French. These experiences, blending cultures of villages far and near, are priceless.

Today, I style my own hair because I have chosen to grow very long dreadlocks, but those early days of redefining myself by putting down the relaxer chemicals full of sodium hydroxide, straightening combs, and smothering grease en route to reclaiming my cultural identity have made an indelible impact on my memory.

A friend of mine, A. J. Johnson, has a very upscale salon called Ajes: The Hair Salon, which started in the village where I live but moved quite a few years ago to downtown Chicago. I have gone to him off and on for many years, and I have brought my children there to have their hair done as well. At Ajes, the clientele is diverse, according to A.J., with an age range typically from nineteen to sixty-five. "We have numerous multiracial clients, a large number of Latino women, career women, conservative people, artists, high fashion models coming in for photo-styling before commercial and magazines shoots," Johnson says. Much of his work comes from a high-profile model client—this diverse clientele is seeking one thing that is growing in importance to the black community—natural hair care.

In an interview at his loft, aglow from an altar of earthy-scented pillar candles, I asked A.J. questions about his sojourn into natural hair care. The quote that stuck with me the most was as follows:

> We hire loc techicians to start folks out with their new locs. We deal with varied texture of really curly hair with ample amounts of conditioner, use color to enhance natural texture, will braid set to emphasize texture. Natural hair is the most versatile. This is what we do.

When I asked what advice he would give someone transitioning from chemical straighteners or flat irons to embracing their natural style, A.J. replied:

> I'd stress the advantages to their hair's health and ease this will bring to their daily regimen (workouts, for example). No burns, less breakage, no reverting [going back], nicer looking hair all around. I would describe the fullness and density they would achieve.

A.J. uses several techniques to help women transition their hair to natural. Today there are many black women in all walks of life and of various ages wearing natural hairstyles, ranging from short cropped hair to full-blown afro puffs, locs, twists, knots, head wraps, semi-head wraps, cornrows, double-strand twists, and everything in between—all gently kissed by an array of African tree medicines, shea butter chief among them.

CAM *and Activism in the Community*

Nzingha Amma Nommo, founder and owner of Afri-Ware, an African-centered bookstore in my village of Oak Park, Illinois, is a grassroots activist of a different sort. Her way is through African-centered books, clothing, and healing tools. Afri-Ware is a store where African oils, resins, minerals, incense, and other natural products coexist in an educational environment, where there are inspirational speakers and motivational books concerned with Afrocentric wellness and our history, health, and politics. According to Nommo,

> We have found that combining African-centered books with natural products fulfills two essential community needs:
>
> >> Reading and seeing about our culture
>
> >> Practicing our culture.
>
> Our ancestral recipes for survival must be lived out through us to preserve our legacies. Reading about our culture grounds us. Practicing our culture binds us . . . the circle is complete.[12]

Bookstores like Afri-Ware can be found across the United States, especially where there are significant African American populations, and the stores are also found elsewhere in the diaspora. African-centered bookstores double as community centers that connect black culture, people, spirituality, enlightenment, political awareness, and wellness.

So What's in It for the Communities?

We must revisit the *Nguzo Sabo* of Kwanzaa and refamiliarize ourselves with several Swahili concepts:

>> *Ujamaa*—**Cooperative Economics:** building and maintaining our own stores, shops, and other businesses to profit, together.

>> *Nia*—**Purpose:** making our collective purpose the building and development of our community. Restoring our people to their traditional greatness.

>> *Kujichagulia*—**To Define Ourselves:** defining ourselves and our customs under our own terms. Naming ourselves, speaking for ourselves visually, spiritually, metaphysically, and culturally.

Socially Responsible Products

Using products or botanical ingredients that have been purchased through fair-trade programs deters the deterioration of local communities and the rich cultural heritage they support. Shea, some types of cocoa (for chocolate and cocoa butter), murumuru, babassu, baobab, sausage tree products, and wild camphor are all wildcrafted by local residents of their respective communities. Purchasing organic, wildcrafted products helps remote communities to gain income opportunities, and it strengthens local economies, sometimes even improving health and literacy projects. This helps indigenous and rural communities retain or build economic independence. It also slows down the economic drive for cutting down trees. The ecosystem is allowed to function naturally, as it has for many years. Through fairly traded products, such as those containing murumuru, the community is rewarded for stewarding trees while the local economy is enhanced.

For example, the river-dwelling population of Marajo stopped cutting down trees, including murumuru palm, once they could generate income from the fruits and fallen seeds of the plants. Professional growth, in harmony with natural resources, is being referred to as "socially responsible entrepreneurship."

Go with the FLO

We must look for FLO labels, especially with African products like chocolate. Fair trade means indigenous people and others from rural village are paid fair market value for their products. In order to be considered fair trade by the FLO (Fairtrade Labelling Organizations International), a product's sale has to lead to decent working conditions, local sustainability, and respect for the local environment and better prices for rural citizens.

I have highlighted some outstanding organizations and individuals working with fair trade, agroforestry, permaculture, health and beauty, and community activism in villages afar and local. There are hundreds of thousands, so this is just a synopsis. Below is a brief summary of some other programs going on in continental Africa and elsewhere in the transatlantic.

INTERNATIONAL COOPERATION:
PAST AND FUTURE OF TREE-CENTERED HOLISTIC PROJECTS

≫ Essential oil has been a Moroccan cottage industry since the seventh century C.E.[13] Equipment and technology has grown obsolete. Morocco, in concert with Canadian researchers supported by the International Development Research Centre (IDRC), is working to develop new stills. Dr. Bachir Benjilali of the Aromatic Plants and Essential Oil Laboratory sees direct progress, as currently hundred of thousands of Moroccan people are employed through the essential oil industry. Professor Benjilali, a former rural villager, is proud to be associated with the first chemical description of verbena oil in the world. *Plantes aromatiques* (Maroc), a project directed by Benjilai and Dr. Belanger of Canada, includes research on chemical compositions, chemotaxonomy, and optimal conditions for exploitation of various herbs and tree medicines.[14]

≫ Students in Free Enterprise (SIFE), a U.S.-led not-for-profit, is working in various West African countries, teaching rural villagers to make soap and botanical cosmetics using local trees and other plants.

≫ Rural Togo, Benin, and Ghana have established distillation technology to extract essential oils under the direction of Vegetal Extracts and Natural Aromas Laboratory et al.

≫ Agribusiness in Sustainable Natural African Plant Products (A-SNAPP) helps rural African communities manufacture tree medicines and other natural products for the international market.[15]

≫ Zambian farmers, in concert with Ecocert in Malawi, have certified organic essential oils. From the forests and savannahs, wildcrafted and organic bee products are also being exported.

≫ Zambili d'Afrique is developing crafts and agricultural products including essential oils, herbs, and spices. As of the year 2000, they have been members of the International Federation of Alternative Trade (IFAT). Zambili products have been inspected by the FLO and the Ethical Trading Initiative (ETI).

≫ Phyto-Trade Africa is a promising African company, representing ethical, organic, sustainable agroforestry products utilizing such trees as mongongo, sausage tree, and baobab from the countries of Botswana, Malawi, Mozambique, Namibia, South Africa, Swaziland, Zambia, and Zimbabwe.

≫ UNIFEM brokered a deal between the women shea butter manufacturers of Burkina Faso and the international natural cosmetic company L'Occitane. Women in Zambia and Zimbabwe organized their own fixed oil and essential oil co-ops. Terra Shea was the first high-profile company, hopefully of many, to buy directly from such co-ops, directly affecting rural economies. This same company also sells quality shea butter and oils from rural communities. In the year 2000 alone, seven million U.S. dollars were earned from sales of shea in Burkina Faso. Parts of Burkina Faso have literacy rates as low as 15 percent, and money from shea sales is used to build literacy among the Burkinabe people, especially the children.[16]

>> In current *Incense land* (Somalia), trade groups wade through politics and tradition to establish the fair trade of frankincense and myrrh, as gender equality through tree tending is sought.

>> An innovative phytotherapy (herbalism) Haitian school featuring nonwestern approaches has been established.[17]

>> The population of Grenada is almost entirely African descended, with 82 percent identified as black and 13 percent biracial, and the rest are native Caribbean groups.[18] Two thousand to twenty-two hundred tons of nutmeg and mace were exported from Grenada in 1994, making it one of their top exports.[19]

>> In 2005 alone, the akee industry of Jamaica was valued at four hundred million dollars. Arils are exported to the United States after undergoing rigorous testing to ensure they are safe for consumption. Traditional distilleries still manufacture bay rum in Jamaica. Allspice and bay rum, grown and processed by Jamaicans, are two more booming economical trees helping the economy of Jamaica.

>> There is a growing grassroots movement within the United States to obtain sufficient medical care for African Americans and to utilize complementary care more. Gullah herbal traditions are being preserved and disseminated.[20] A growing number of black people are embracing traditional African religions (which feature herbalism), and reconnecting to Egyptian spirituality.

In Closing

Trees are vital to the everyday life of many communities, large and small, around Mother Earth. African people especially are dependent on their unique holistic medicines, the economic opportunities they provide, and their spiritual connection to deity as well as their important role in the community. We are awed by the commanding yet mysterious presence of trees, rich with mystical and metaphysical qualities and great potential.

As members of one of the oldest continuous cultures on the face of the earth, people of African descent have a significant role in the stewardship of the trees and the forest culture that has been sustained. We also have a special opportunity to share the little-known story of our lives within the Sacred Wood with countless others. I look forward to the conversation continuing with those willing to listen, share, and pay it forward.

Resources and Organizations

I suggest beginning in some small way to make a change in a personal way and developing out from there. This would include:

≫ Try out the herbs, recipes, rituals, and alternate ways of preparing and thinking about food presented here.

≫ Experiment with developing your own fresh homemade juices and drinks.

≫ Collect and adapt family or regional recipes.

≫ Learn about your culture, whether regional, ethnic, or spirit.

≫ Reach out to begin or reinforce holistic programs in your community.

≫ Work to educate others, working through schools, community centers, and co-ops.

≫ Support local concerns that promote fair trade, sustainability, and wholesome living.

≫ Start an ongoing participatory group with like minded people—this can be an online group such as www.meetup.com.

≫ Examine the land rights and land tenure activity as well as fair and equitable housing where you live.

≫ Support local environmental initiatives that impact the environment including ordinances, laws, conservatories, reserves, forest preserves, and environmental protection organizations.

≫ Support local growing initiatives, local holistic health facilities, shops, farmers markets, co-ops, concerns, and botanical products.

≫ Find a meaningful way to intersect mind, body, and spirit—this can be through exercise, meditation, spiritual activity, or daily affirmations.

Whatever you choose to do on a local level, sharing should be a central aspect.

Nationally and internationally there are many organizations, particularly NGOs dedicated to various ways of strengthening indigenous culture and sustainable life style. You are sure to find organizations that speak to your personality. Here are a few organizations either mentioned in the book or which have informed it in one way or another, which you may wish to contact to support, or for further information:

Africa Recovery

Africa Recovery Room S-931, United Nations, New York 10017 USA

Phone: (212) 963-6857; Fax: (212) 963-4556

E-mail: africa_recovery@un.org

Africa Recovery faces issues concerning African women farmers.

A-SNAPP: Agribusiness in Sustainable Natural African Plant Products

c/o Herb Research Foundation, 1007 Pearl St. Suite 200, Boulder, CO USA 80302

American Botanical Council can be reached at this same address. American Botanical Council produces a general interest herbal magazine, a professional journal, and has the German E Commission herbal monographs cited in this book available for purchase.

Black Midwives

www.blackmidwives.org

This organization seeks to reduce black infant mortality, instill natural midwife-led childbirth, preserve the black granny midwife tradition, and support holistic health in the community.

Food First

www.foodfirst.org

Institute for Food and Development Policy, 398 60th St., Oakland, CA 94618

Phone: (510) 654-4400

Greenbelt Movement (GBM)

www.greenbeltmovement.org

P.O. Box 67545, Nairobi, Kenya

Phone: +254 20 573057 571523

Langata Training Centre: +254 20 891679

E-mail: gbm@wananchi.com

Gullah/Geechee Sea Island Coalition Homebase

Post Office Box 1207, St. Helena Island SC 29920

Phone: (843) 838-1171

This membership organization preserves and maintains Gullah culture of the Lowcountry.

Historic Seeds

www.historictrees.org

American Forests' Historic Tree Nursery

8701 Old Kings Road,

Jacksonville, FL, 32219

Phone: (800) 320-8733

International Development Research Centre
Dr. Honore Kossi Koumaglo,
Vegetal Extracts and Natural Aromas Laboratory,
(LEVAN) Department of Sciences,
University of Benin, PO Box 1515, Lome Togo
E-mail: hkoumagl@syfed.tg.refer.org

Dr. Koumaglo can be contacted regarding African essential oil research and development projects.

Institut agronomique et veterinaire Hassan II
Professor Bachir Benjilali, PO Box 6202, Rabat-Instituts, Morocco

Agriculture Canada Research Centre
Andre Belanger, 430 Gouin Blvd.
St-Jean-sur-Richelieu, Quebec J3B 6Z8

National Campaign for Sustainable Agriculture
P.O. Box 396, Pine Bush, NY, 12566
Phone: (845) 744-8448; Fax: (845) 744-8477

OXFAM International
Make Trade Fair Campaign
www.maketradefair.com

Students in Free Enterprise (SIFE)
1959 East Kerr Street Springfield, MO
USA 65803-4775

SIFE works toward establishing, building, and maintaining fair-trade initiatives in Africa and elsewhere, such as the soapmaking project at University Ghana, Legon, featured in this book.

Supporting Black (American) Farmers
Economic Human Rights:
The Time Has Come! Campaign
www.foodfirst.org
Food First, 398 60th Street, Oakland CA 94618
Phone: (510) 654-4400

Federation of Southern Cooperatives
2769 Church Street, Eastpoint GA 30344
Phone: (404) 765-0991

Black Farmers and Agriculturalists Association
PO Box 597, Buena Vista GA 31803

Pan American Health Organization
www.paho.org
525 23rd Street, NW. Washington, D.C. 20037
Phone: (202) 974-3305; Fax: (202) 974-3623
E-mail: library@paho.org

UNAIDS
www.unaids.org
Donor Relations 20, Avenue Appia, CH-1211
Geneva 27
Switzerland

This international organization works with HIV/AIDS around the world.

UNIFEM
304 E. 45th Street, 15th Floor,
New York, NY, 10017
West African Contact: Florence Butegwa
11 Oyinkan Abayomi Drive, Ikoyi, Lagos, Nigeria

This United Nations organization helps women with various projects and initiatives.

United Plant Savers
P.O. Box 400 E. Barre, VT 05649
Phone: (802)-479-9825; Fax: (802) 476-3722
E-mail: info@unitedplantsavers.org

Zambili d'Afrique
PO Box 38540, Lusaka, Zambia
E-mail: zagric@zambili.co.zm

Contact this organization for more information on the Zambian women' s project with essential oils and African crafts.

Appendix A

RESOURCES

ESSENTIAL OILS AND HYDROSOLS

Liberty Natural Products, Inc.
www.libertynatural.com
8120 SE Stark St. Portland, OR 97215
Phone: (503) 256-1227

Carnation absolute, rose otto/attar of roses, champa oil, quality frankincense, myrrh, bamboo charcoal, essential oils at descent prices considering the preciousness of rare oils.

EXOTIC OILS AND INCENSE SUPPLIES

Scents of Earth
www.scents-of-earth/info.html
PO Box 859, Sun City, CA 92586
Phone: (800) 323-8159
E-mail: info@scents-of-earth.com

Sells quality lotus oils, sandalwood, attars, and prayer incense.

White Lotus Aromatics
www.whitelotusaromatics.com
Christopher McMahon, 801 Park Way,
El Cerrito, CA 94530
 E-mail: somanth@aol.com

Oils from India including a variety of lotus oils, attars, ruhs, and incense as well.

HENNA

One of the best sources of henna information is organized by the scholar Catherine Cartwright-Jones at www.mehandi.com. Her site features various henna pattern and henna history books (Henna Page Productions/Tap Dancing Lizard) and information on suppliers, as well as recipes and history.

HERBS AND PLANTS BY MAIL ORDER

Clifton Flower and Garden Center
1254 W. Olive, Porterville, CA 93257

Sells a variety of fragrant plants by mail order including citrus trees; types discussed in this book.

Richters Herb Specialists,
www.richters.com

Books on tulsi and other species of plants, as well as numerous other aromatic plants and seeds.

San Francisco Herb Co.
250 14th St., San Francisco, CA 94103-2420
Phone: (415) 861-7174

HOODOO BOOKS AND SUPPLIES

Lucky Mojo Curio Catalog
www.luckymojo.com
6632 Kovey Road, Forestville, CA 95436

Hoodoo books, supplies, incenses, and powders.

PACKAGING/BOTTLES AND JARS

Reuse/Recycle

The first option is to sterilize, reuse, and thereby recycle your own bottles.

Shampoo and conditioner bottles come in handy for homemade hair care products.

Dish soap bottles are handy for home cleaning products.

A vinegar rinse will get rid of previous smells and chemicals.

Baby food and pasta sauce jars are handy for quick storage.

Ziploc or other sturdy plastic bags come in handy for temporary storage of dried botanicals.

Packaging Companies

Papermart
www.papermart.com
5361 Alexander Street, Los Angeles, CA 90040
Phone: (800) 745-8800

Carries professional quality plastic bags, paper bags, containers, packaging for soap, gift boxes, muslin bags, sachets, raffia, ribbon, and shipping materials.

Sunburst Bottle Company
www.sunburstbottle.com
4500 Beloit Drive, Sacramento, CA 95838
Phone: (916) 929-4500; Fax: (916) 929-3604
E-mail: info@sunburstbottle.com

Spray top, brown and cobalt glass bottles, powder/shaker packaging, and fancy decorative bottles for herbal blends and botanical crafts.

PREPARED PRODUCTS

Africas Garden
www.africasgarden.com
Phone: (888) 264-0888; Fax: (310) 274-4006;
E-mail: Customerservice@africasgarden.com

Moringa and other African oils, Egyptian aromatherapy products, African sea sponge.

Gardener's Supply Company
Gardener's Supply Company, 128 Intervale Road, Burlington, VT 05401
Phone: (888) 833-1412; Fax: (800) 551-6712
E-mail: info@gardeners.com

Lavender body wrap, mitts, or gloves to use in Cocoa Body Butter Bliss Treatment.

L'Occitane en Provence
www.loccitane.com

Carries shea butter products purchased directly from African women through co-ops. International natural product company has lotus, neroli, magnolia, sandalwood, orange, life everlasting, patchouli, shea, and other products discussed in this book.

Moon Garden Creations
Moon Garden Creations, 1529 George Ave, Jefferson City, TN, 37760
E-mail WinterJKD@aol.com

Woman-owned small business founded by Jannette Giles-Hypes features a heavenly healing body butter that contains shea, mango, and cocoa butter among other wholesome oils.

Terra Shea Organics African Shea Butter Company
www.africansheabuttercompany.com
8400-C Hilltop Rd, Fairfax, VA 22031
Phone: (877) 427-6627
E-mail: Sales@africansheabuttercompany.com

Black soap, argun oil, Rhassoul mud, shea butters, black seed oil, and baobab oil.

SOAPMAKING AND NATURAL HOME CLEANING PRODUCTS

Rainbow Meadow
www.rainbowmeadow.com

A woman-owned Internet company providing soapmaking supplies.

Sunfeather Soap Company
www.sunsoap.com
1551 Hwy 72, Potsdam NY 13676
Phone: (315) 265-3648; Fax: (315) 265-2902
E-mail: sunsoap@sunsoap.com

A woman-owned business founded by Sandy Maine with soapmaking and natural home-cleaning supplies, butters, oils, molds, and chocolate fragrance oil.

Wholesale Supplies Plus, Inc.
www.wholesalesuppliesplus.com
13390 York Road, Unit G,
North Royalton, OH, 44133
E-mail: soaporder@aol.com

Sells essential oils, carrier oils, MP soap blocks, bottles, jars, and other packaging.

STATUARY: EGYPTIAN, HINDU, YORUBA, SAINTS

Check out your local botanicas, galleries, and shops first. African, Gullah, and Caribbean artists often attend local street fairs, arts and crafts fairs, and trade shows.

Sacred Source
www.sacredsource.com
P.O. Box 163WW, Crozet, VA 22932
Phone: (800) 290-6203; Fax: (434) 823-7665

AFRICAN AND HAITIAN ART

RIDGE ART
 www.ridgeart.com
21 Harrison Street, Oak Park, IL 60304

Appendix B

STUDY AND APPRENTICESHIPS

LATIN AMERICA AND NORTH AFRICA

Body, Mind, Spirit Journeys to Costa Rica and Egyptian Pyramids
Sacred Journey Tours and Mystery School
www.soulmatters.com
E-mail: insite@soulmatters.com
Facilitated by Constance S. Rodriguez, Ph.D.

SOUTH AFRICA

ecoAfrica Travel (Pty) Ltd.
www.ecoBotswana.com, www.ecoKruger.com,
www.ecoAfrica.com
Stellenbosch, South Africa
Phone: +27 21 809 2180; Fax: +27 21 809 2189

Arranges experiences with South African Sangoma healers and herbalists. Can arrange South African herb/wildlife study tour, safari, individual or group experiences, and eco-tours.

CARIBBEAN/HAITI; EAST AND WEST AFRICA

See Ridge Art listing on page 211.

The Aromatic Plant Project
www.aromaticplantproject.com
PO Box 225336, San Francisco, CA 94122-5336

Founded by aromatherapist Jeanne Rose; supplies information regarding hydrosol workshops, aromatic plants, with newsletter and seasonal recipes.

Handmade Beauty Network
www.handmadebeauty.com

African American president Donna Marie Cole, Esq., of this company offers a newsletter, membership, fellowship, and recipes for botanical cosmetics and holistic living.

Heal Thyself Natural Living Center
www.queenafuaonline.com
106 Kingston Avenue, Brooklyn, NY, 11213
Phone: (718) 221-HEAL

Clay products, fasting and cleansing kits, books, information, training, and consultation dedicated to Khemetian health practices.

Ifa Foundation of North America
http://ifafoundation.org
E-mail: iyanifa@cfl.rr.com

Workshops and readings; has a college, Babalawo training, and bookstore.

Stephanie Rose Bird is an artist, exhibiting nature-inspired and floral paintings, two lines of products, and workshops and classes in various locations. Contact through the publisher.

In closing, I hope you will not find the prospect of reaching out to explore the themes in this book daunting. Remember the words of Lao Tzu: *A journey of a thousand miles begins with a single step.*

Notes

INTRODUCTION

1. *Dictionary of American Family Names* (Oxford University Press). www.ancestry.com (accessed December 10, 2007).

2. Mitchell, Faith, *Hoodoo Medicine: Gullah Herbal Remedies* (Columbia, SC: Summerhouse Press, 1999).

3. Thompson, Robert Farris, *Flash of the Spirit: African and Afro-American Art and Philosophy* (New York: Random House, 1989), 138–139.

4. Ibid.

5. Mitchell, *Hoodoo Medicine.*

6. Integrative Medicine Communications, "Pine," *The Complete German Commission E Monographs: Therapeutic Guide to Herbal Medicines* (Austin, TX: American Botanic Council, 1988).

7. McCormick, Jack, "The Vegetation of the New Jersey Pine Barrens," in *Pine Barrens: Ecosystem and Landscape*, ed. Forman, Richard T. T. (New Brunswick, NJ: Rutgers, State University Press, 1998).

8. Wall, Carly, *The Scented Veil: Using Scent to Awaken the Soul* (Virginia Beach, VA: ARE Press, 2002).

CHAPTER 1

1. Diallo, Yaya, *The Healing Drum of Africa* (Rochester, VT: Destiny Books, 1989), 61.

2. Ibid., 20–21.

3. Ibid., 21.

4. Asare, Edmund, "Traditional Knowledge in Forest Conservation: Case Study of the Malshegu Community in Ghana" (paper), Tampere Poytechnic, Finland.

5. Peterson, Karen, "Seacology Helps Conserve Medicinal Plants of Madagascar," *Journal of the American Botanical Council* 65 (2005): 20.

6. Githetho, Anthony N., "Sacred Land Film Project: The Sacred Mijikenda Kaya Forests of Coastal Kenya and Biodiversity Conservation" (paper): 27–35.

7. Fett, Sharla M., *Working Cures: Healing, Health, and Power on Southern Slave Plantations* (Chapel Hill, NC: University of North Carolina, 2002), 8.

8. Bird, Stephanie, *Sticks, Stones, Roots and Bones: Hoodoo, Mojo and Conjuring with Herbs* (St. Paul, MN: Llewellyn, 2004), 31–34.

9. Packenham, T., *Remarkable Trees of the World* (New York and London: W. W. Norton & Company, 2003), 142.

CHAPTER 2

1. LaGamma, Alisa, and John Pemberton, *Oracle: African Art and Rituals of Divination* (New York: HNA Books, 2000).

2. Makinde, M. A., *African Philosophy, Culture, and Traditional Medicine* (Athens, OH: Ohio University Center for International Studies, Africa Series Number 53, 1988), 88.

3. Makinde, *African Philosophy*, 43; Olmos, Margarite Fernandez, and Lizabeth Paravisini-Gebert, *Sacred Possessions: Voodoo, Santeria, Obeah and the Caribbean* (New Brunswick, NJ: Rutgers University Press, 1997), 50.

4. Olmos, *Sacred Possessions*, 49–51.

5. Thompson, *Flash of the Spirit*, 42.

6. Ibid., 43.

7. LaGamma, *Art and Oracle*, 46.

8. Ibid.

9. Stroup, Thomas, "A Charm from North Carolina and The Merchant of Venice, II, vii, 75," *Journal of American Folklore* 49 (1936), 266.

10. Alleyne, Mervyn C., and Arvilla Payne-Jackson, *Jamaican Folk Medicine: A Source of Healing* (Kingston, Jamaica: University of the West Indies Press, 2004), 105–111.

11. Diallo, Yaya, and Hall, Mitchell, *The Healing Drum: African Wisdom Teachings* (Rochester, VT: Destiny Books, 1989), 80.

12. Djembe and Mande Music Page/Review Section (revised February 11, 1999), http://tcd.freehosting.net/djembemande/jelicds.html (accessed December 11, 2008).

13. Doumbia, A., and B. Doumbia, *The Way of the Elders: West African Spirituality and Tradition* (St. Paul, MN: Llewellyn Worldwide, 2004), 100–101.

14. *Encyclopaedia Britannica*, www.britannica.com (last accessed January 20, 2008); "Mali," *Funk & Wagnalls New Encyclopedia* (2006).

15. "Mali," *Funk & Wagnalls New Encyclopedia* (2006), 97.

16. *Jaliology*. Xenophile XENO 4036; The Gambia, Senegal.

17. Grime, William Ed, *Ethno-Botany of the Black Americans* (Algonac, MI: Reference Publications, 1979), 12–13.

18. Scarborough, 101.

19. Grime, William Ed, *Ethno-Botany of the Black Americans* (Algonac, MI: Reference Publications, 1979), 137–138.

20. Ibid.

CHAPTER 3

1. Edwards, Victoria H., *The Aromatherapy Companion: Medicinal Uses/Ayurvedic Healing/ Body-Care Blends/Perfumes and Scents/ Emotional Health and Well-Being* (North Adams, MA: Storey Books, 1999), 7.

2. Manniche, L., *An Ancient Egyptian Herbal* (Great Britain: British Museum Press and the University of Texas Press, 1989), 10–12.

3. Edwards, *The Aromatherapy Companion*, 7–8.

4. Manniche, *Sacred Luxuries: Fragrance, Aromatherapy and Cosmetics in Ancient Egypt* (Ithaca, NY: Cornell University Press, 1999), 10–12.

5. Ibid., 114.

6. Doumbia, Adama, and Naomi Doumbia, *The Way of the Elders: West African Spirituality and Tradition* (St. Paul, MN: Llewellyn Worldwide., 2004), 91.

7. Ibid., 90.

8. Manniche, *An Ancient Egyptian Herbal*, 13.

9. Ibid., 76–77.

10. Williams, Larry, and Charles S. Finch, "The Great Queens of Ethiopia" in *Civilizations* 6:1 (New Brunswick & London: Transaction Publishers, 2002), 12.

11. Karade, "Pre-Historic Nations," 61.

12. Williams, "The Great Queen of Ethiopia," 13.

13. Rashidi, R., "African Goddesses," in *Civilizations* 6:1 (New Brunswick & London: Transaction Publishers, 2002), 72.

14. Redd, D., "Hatsheput," in *Black Women in Antiquity* (New Brunswick & London: Transaction Publishers, 2002), 213.

15. Davidson, Basil, *The Lost Cities of Africa* (Boston: Little, Brown, 1959), 60.

16. Omoleya, Michael, *Certificate History of Nigeria* (London & Lagos: Longman Group, 1986), 15.

17. Karade, "Pre-Historic Nations," 3.

18. Alleyne and Payne-Jackson, *Jamaican Folk Medicine*, 52–56.

19. E. Paravisini-Gebert and M. Fernandez Olmos, *Creole Religions of the Caribbean: An Introduction from Vodou and Santeria to Obeah and Espiritismo* (New York: New York University Press, 2003).

20. Some, Malidoma Patrice, *The Healing Wisdom of Africa: Finding Life Purpose Through Nature, Ritual, and Community* (New York: Putnam Tarcher, 1999), 263.

21. Katz, R., *Boiling Energy: Community Healing Among the Kalahari Kung* (Cambridge, MA: Harvard University Press, 1982), 251.

22. "Kalahari Desert—The Last Paradise on Earth: The People, Plants and Animals of the Kalahari," http://abbott-infotech.co.za/index-kalahari.html.

23. "Tribes of the Kalahari," http://abbott-infotech.co.za/tribes%20in%20the%20kalahari.html (accessed December 15, 2007).

24. Katz, *Boiling Energy*.

25. Ibid., 18.

26. "Kalahari Desert—The Last Paradise on Earth."

27. Katz, *Boiling Energy*, 93.

28. Marshall, L., *!Kung Bushman Religious Beliefs* (*Africa*, no. 32, 1962), 246.

29. Katz, *Boiling Energy*, 21, 23, 25.

CHAPTER 4

1. Voeks, Robert, *Sacred Leaves of Candomblé* (Austin, TX: University of Texas Press, 1997), 160–161.

2. Abbiw, *Useful Plants of Ghana*.

3. Plants for Clean Air Council, http://www.zone10.com/tech/NASA/Fyh.htm (accessed April 23, 2008).

4. Nickens, T. E., "Saving the Spirit Trees," www.americanforests.org, 2003 fall feature (accessed December 31, 2007).

5. Scheub, Harold, *A Dictionary of African Mythology: The Mythmaker as Storyteller* (Oxford and New York: Oxford University Press, 2000), 124–125.

6. Abbiw, *Useful Plants of Ghana*, 171.

7. Nickens, Edward, "Saving the Spirit Trees," www.americanforests.org, 2003 fall feature (accessed December 31, 2007).

8. Von Maydell, 1986

9. Allen, O. N., and E. K. Allen, *The Leguminosae: A Source Book of Characteristics, Uses and Nodulation* (Madison, WI: University of Wisconsin Press, 1981).

10. Nickens, Edward, *Saving Spirit Trees* (Washington, DC: American Forests, 2007), www.americanforests.org (last accessed December 31, 2007).

11. Baobab Fact Sheet, International Centre for Underutilized Crops, 2003.

12. PhytoTrade Africa, 2003. www.phytotradeafrica.com (last accessed February 10, 2009).

13. Abbiw, *Useful Plants of Ghana*, 127.

14. Baobab Fact Sheet.

15. Nickens, *Saving Spirit Trees.*

16. Buckley, A. D., *Yoruba Medicine* (New York: Athelia Henrietta Press, 1997), 225.

17. LaGamma, *Art and Oracle*, 28.

18. Little, K. L., *The Mende of Sierra Leone* (London: Routledge and Kegan Paul, 1951), 240.

19. Alldridge, T. J., *The Sherbro and Its Hinterland* (London: MacMillan and Co., 1901), 147–148.

20. Buckley, *Yoruba Medicine*, 209.

21. Ibid., 225.

22. Ibid., 209.

23. Almquist, Alden, "Divination and the Hunt in Pagibeti Ideology," in *African Divination Systems: Ways of Knowing* (Bloomington, IN:Indiana University Press, 1991).

24. Ibid.

25. Ibid., 27.

26. For the younger set, ages four through eight: Onyefulu, I., *Ebele's Favorite: A Book of African Games* (London, England: Frances Lincoln Press, 2000), featuring ten traditional Nigerian games; Zaslavsky, C., *Africa Counts: Number and Pattern in African Cultures* (Chicago: Lawrence Hill Books; 1999) for adults to teach children about African games and counting systems.

27. Zaslavsky, C., *Africa Counts: Number and Pattern in African Cultures* (Chicago: Lawrence Hill Books; 1999).

CHAPTER 5

1. Turnbull, Colin, *The Forest People: A Study of the Pygmies of the Congo* (New York: Simon & Schuster, 1961), 13.

2. Mack, C. K., and D. Mack, *A Field Guide to Demons, Fairies, Fallen Angels, and Other Subversive Spirits* (New York: Henry Holt, Inc., 1998), 63.

3. Guerry, V., *Life with the Baoule*, trans. Nora Hodges (Washington, DC: Three Continents Press, 1975), 138–44.

4. Mack, *A Field Guide to Demons*, 102–103.

5. Ibid., 123–124.

6. Ibid., 114–115.

7. Angelique, Madrina, Erzulie's AuthenticVoudou, http://www.erzulies.com/site/articles/view/8 (accessed March 6, 2008).

8. Ibid.

9. LaGamma, *Art and Oracle*, 44–45.

10. Thompson, R., *Black Gods and Kings* (Los Angeles: UCLA Flower Museum of Cultural History, 1976), 99.

11. Turnbull, *The Forest People*.

12. Ibid.

13. Ibid.

14. www.ghana.co.uk/history/fashion/adrinka_adinka symblos.htm (last accessed December 17, 2007).

15. www.risc.org.uk/bogolan/index.htm (last accessed December 17, 2007).

16. Turnbull, *The Forest People*, 54

17. Fontenot, W., *Secret Doctors: Ethnomedicines of African Americans* (Westport, CT: Bergin & Garvey, 1994).

18. Scott, G., *Headwraps: A Global Journey* (Cambridge, MA: Perseus Books and New York: Public Affairs Books, 2003), 184.

19. Ibid., 13.

20. Ibid., 178.

21. Fontenot, *Secret Doctors*, 117.

22. Thompson, *Flash of the Spirit*, 68.

23. Fontenot, *Secret Doctors*, 71.

24. Drewal, H. J., "Arts and Divination Among the Yoruba: Design and Myth," *African Journal* 14: 2–3 (1987), 42.

25. Makinde, *African Philosophy, Cultures, and Traditional Medicine*.

26. Schildkrout, E., and C. A. Keim, *African Reflections* (exhibition catalog) (New York: American Museum of Natural History, 1990), 174–178.

27. Ibid., 185.

28. Fontenot, *Secret Doctors*, 115.

29. Moore, K., "Seed Jewelry: Seeds Used as Beads: Facts and Folkore," *Plantlore* 6 (1982): 19–27.

30. *From My People—400 Years of African American Folklore* Cumber Dance, Daryl (ed). (NY: W.W. Norton & Company, 2002).

CHAPTER 6

1. Makinde, *African Philosophy, Culture, and Traditional Medicine*, 92.

2. Thompson, *Flash of the Spirit*, 9.

3. Feeley-Harnik, G., "Cloth and the Creation of Ancestors in Madagascar," in Weiner, A., and J. Schneider (eds.), *Cloth and Human Experience* (Chicago, IL: University of Chicago Press).

4. http://library.thinkquest.org/27209/animal.htm (last accessed December 17, 2007).

5. Katz, R., *Community Healing Among the Kalahari Kung* (Cambridge, MA: Harvard University Press, 1982), 93.

6. Biesele, M., *Folklore and Ritual of !Kung Hunter-Gatherers*, 2 vols. (doctoral dissertation) (Cambridge, MA: Harvard University, 1975).

7. Katz, R., *Community Healing Among the Kalahari Kung* (Cambridge, MA: Harvard University Press, 1982), 97.

8. Biesele, *Folklore and Ritual of !Kung Hunter-Gatherers*.

CHAPTER 7

1. Rulangaranga, Z.K. (1989) Some Important Indigenous Medicinal and Aromatic Plants in the Wild Flora of Tanzania Mainland. Tropical Forest Action Plan, Working Paper 24. Tanzania: Ministry of Lands, Natural Resources and Tourism, Dar es Salaam; EROS Data Centre, International Program, Cape Chestnut Tree, 2003; Kew, 1984. Royal Botanic Gardens. Forage and Browse Plants for Arid and Semi-Arid Africa. International Board for Genetic Resources: Royal Botanic Gardens.

2. EROS Data Centre, International Program, Cape Chestnut Tree, 2003

3. Manniche, *An Ancient Egyptian Herbal*, 122–123.

4. Ibid.

5. Staff Writer, "Jatropha Oil, Women's Fuel Project," *Arusha Times*, September 9, 2002.

6. www.jatrophabiodiesel.org/aboutJatrophaPlant.php?_divid=menu1.

7. Bremness, L., *A Fragrant Herbal: Enhancing Your Life with Aromatic Herbs and Essential Oils* (New York: Little, Brown & Co., 1998), 230; "Nutmeg and Mace (*Myristica fragrans*)," www.uni-graz.at/~Katzer/engl/Myri_fra.html (last accessed January 8, 2008); Bremness, *A Fragrant Herbal*, 230.

8. "Nutmeg and Mace," www.fao.org/docrep/v4084e/v4084eOb.htm (last accessed January 8, 2008); Central Intelligence Agency, "Grenada," in *The World Fact Book*, www.cia.gov/library/publications/the-world-factbook/print/gj.html (last updated and accessed January 8, 2008); www.fao.org/docrep/v4084e/v4084eOb.htm (last accessed January 8, 2008).

9. Bremness, *A Fragrant Herbal*, 230.

10. www.fao.org/docrep/v4084e/v4084eOb.htm (last accessed January 8, 2008).

11. Neem Foundation, 1997. "The Neem Tree an Introduction and History," www.neemfoundation.org (last accessed February 4, 2009).

12. Kimathi, H., "Neem: The Wonder Tree." CAHNET News 2003.

13. Ibid.

CHAPTER 8

1. Schildkrout, E., and C. A. Keim, *African Reflections* (exhibition catalog) (New York: American Museum of Natural History, 1990): 173, 177, 185–187.

2. Abbiw, *Useful Plants of Ghana*, 44–45.

3. Maathai, Wangari, *The Greenbelt Movement,* revised edition (New York: Lantern Books, 2003).

4. Abbiw, *Useful Plants of Ghana*, 44–45.

5. Dooley, Elizabeth B. K., *Puerto Rican Cookbook* (Richmond, VA: Dietz Press, 1948), 99–100.

6. Carper, Jean, *Food: Your Miracle Medicine* (New York: Harper Collins Publishers, 1993), 102–103.

7. Abbiw, *Useful Plants of Ghana*, 30.

8. Carper, *Food*, 102–103.

9. Abbiw, *Useful Plants of Ghana*, 44.

10. Carper, *Food*, 338, 405; Dooley, *Puerto Rican Cookbook,* 125–126.

11. Davidson, A., and C. Knox, *Fruit—A Connoisseur's Guide and Cookbook* (New York, NY: Simon and Schuster, 1991).

12. Dweck, A. C., "Ethnobotanical Plants from Africa, part II," *Cosmetics and Toiletries* magazine, (Black Medicare Ltd: Iltshire, UK, 2001).

13. Abbiw, *Useful Plants of Ghana*, 44.

14. Dweck, "Ethnobotanical Plants from Africa, part II."

15. Ibid.

16. Roodt, Veronica, "Kigelia Africana," *Shell Field Guide to the Common Trees of the Okavango Delta and Moremi Game Reserve* (Gaborone, Botswana: Shell Oil Botswana, 1992).

17. "The Strange Sausage Tree," *Encounter South Africa,* www.encounter.co.za/article/66htm (accessed December 21, 2007).

18. Houghton, P., et al., "Activity of extracts of Kigelia pinnata against melanoma and renal carcinoma cell lines," *Planta Medica* 60: 5 (1994), 430–433.

19. Abbiw, *Useful Plants of Ghana.*

20. "Sausage Trees at PhytoTrade Africa."

21. Abbiw, *Useful Plants of Ghana*, 149, 163–164.

22. Morton, J., "Breadfruit," in *Fruits of Warm Climates* (Miami, FL: Julia J. Morton, 1987), http://www.hort.purdue.edu/newcrop/morton/breadfruit.html (accessed January 5, 2008).

23. Morton, J., "Breadfruit," in *Fruits of Warm Climates*; Breadfruit Institute, National Tropical Botanical Garden, 2007, www.ntbg.org/breadfruit/uses/ (last accessed January 4, 2008).

24. Pinto, A. C. de Q., and M. C. R. Cordeiro, S. R. M. de Andrade, F. R. Ferreira, H. A. de C. Filgueiras, R. E. Alves, and D. E. Kinpara, "Annona Species," International Centre of Underutilized Crops, Southampton, U.K. (2005).

25. Alleyne and Payne-Jackson, *Jamaican Folk Medicine*, 154–155, 161.

26. Pinto et al., "Annona Species."

27. Ibid.

28. Alleyne and Payne-Jackson, *Jamaican Folk Medicine*, 164.

29. Abbiw, *Useful Plants of Ghana*, 45.

30. Pinto et al., "Annona Species."

31. Ibid.

32. Ibid.

33. Ibid.

34. Ibid.

35. Department of Chemistry, University of West Indies, Lancashire, Kingston 7, Jamaica (1994), http://wwwchem.uwimona.edu.jm/chrl.html (updated and accessed February 10, 2009).

36. "Herbs, Spices and Flavorings," http://en.wikipedia.org/wiki/Allspice (last modified and accessed January 8, 2008).

37. Worwood, V. A., *The Fragrant Heavens* (Novato, CA: New World Library, 1991), 403.

38. Bremness, *A Fragrant Herbal*, 235.

39. Morton, "Pomegranate."

40. Ibid.

41. Ibid.

42. Boulos, L. *Medical Plants of North America.* Algonac, MI: Reference Publications, Inc., 1983:149–150.

43. Brown, D. J., "Pomegranate Juice Improves Carotid Artery Health and Lowers Blood Pressure in Patients with Carotid Artery Stenosis" (clinical update) *Herbal Gram: The Journal of the American Botanical Council* 65 (2005): 28–30.

44. Lust, John, *The Herb Book* (New York: Bantam Books, 1974), 303–304.

45. Carper, *Food*, 410.

46. American Botanical Council, "Herbal Gram," Issue 48 (Austin, Texas, 2000), 10.

47. Morton, Julia F., "Orange" in *Fruits of Warm Climates* (Miami, FL: Julia F. Morton, 1987), 134–143, www.hort.purdue.edu/newcrop/morton/orange.html (last accessed January 18, 2008).

48. Ibid.

49. Ibid.

50. Ibid., 104.

51. Ibid.

52. Bremness, *A Fragrant Herbal*, 214.

CHAPTER 9

1. Bremness, *A Fragrant Herbal*, 169.

2. Abbiw, *Useful Plants of Ghana*.

3. National Audubon Society, *Field Guide to Trees of the Eastern Region* (New York: Alfred Knopf, 1980), 506–507.

4. Bremness, A *Fragrant Herbal*, 211.

5. Ibid.

6. Ibid., 213–214.

7. Manniche, *An Ancient Egyptian Herbal*, 88–89.

8. Ibid.

9. Lust, *The Herb Book*, 263.

10. Trudge, C., *The Tree* (New York: Crown Publishers, 2006), 217.

11. Worwood, *The Fragrant Heavens*, 77.

12. Wall, *The Scented Veil*, 111–112.

13. www.celestialtides.com (Last accessed February 11, 2009), *Celestial Tides*, 2003; Duke, J. A., *Herbs of the Bible: 2000 Years of Plant Medicine* (Loveland, CO: Interweave Press), 1990; Abbiw, *Useful Plants of Ghana*.

14. Illes, Judika, *Earth Mother Magic* (Gloucester, MA: Fairwinds Press, 2001), 38; Duke, *Herbs of the Bible*.

15. McIntyre, Anne, *The Complete Woman's Herbal* (New York: Henry Holt, 1994), 42, 150.

16. Raintree Nutrition, Inc., *Ethnomedical Information on Pau d'Arco* (Carson City, NV: Raintree Nutrition, www.rain-tree.com/paudarco.htm (last accessed January 8, 2008).

17. Ibid.

18. "Complementary and Alternative Therapies for Cancer Patients," University of California, San Diego (La Jolla, CA), www.rain-tree.com (last accessed January 8, 2008).

19. Ibid.

20. Lust, *The Herb Book*, 486.

21. Worwood, *The Fragrant Heavens*, 77.

22. Fett, *Working Cures*, 64.

23. Puckett, Newbell Niles, *Folk Beliefs of the Southern Negro* (Montclair, NJ: Patterson Smith, 1968), 386; Mitchell, *Hoodoo Medicine*, 51.

CHAPTER 10

1. hooks, bell, *Sisters of the Yam* (New York: South End Press; Gloria Watkins, 1993), 180.

2. Trudge, *The Tree*, 140.

3. Ibid., 146.

4. Ibid., 140.

5. Abbiw, 68.

6. Trudge, *The Tree*, 143.[S/B 353]

7. Buckley, *Yoruba Medicine*, 124.

8. Ibid., 108–111.

9. Darish, P., "Dressing for the Next Life: Raffia Textile Production and Use Among the Kuba of Zaire," in *Cloth and Human Experience*, eds. Weiner, A., and J. Schneider, (Wenner-Gren Foundation for Anthropological Research, Washington, DC: Smithsonian, 1989), 118.

10. Linné (1734) cited in Keaney, T.H. (1906): "Date varieties and Date Culture in Tunis." Washington, U.S.D.A; Bureau of Plant Industry, Bulletin No. 92.

11. Pliny, C. (1489): The elder. Trans. Historia naturale, Book XIII, cap. iii, 3 columns on the palmae. Translated into Italian by Cristofore Landioro Fiorentino and published by Bartolamio de Zani de Portesio; Van Zyl, H.J. (1983): "Date Cultivation in South Africa." Information Bulletin No. 504; Compiled by the Fruit and Fruit Technology Research Institute, Department of Agriculture, Stellenbosch, RSA. 26pp.

12. Popenoe, W. (1938): "The Date." Ch. 6. in: *Manual of tropical and subtropical fruits.* New-York: The Mcmillan Company.

13. Dowson, V.H.W. (1982): "Date production and protection with special reference to North Africa and the Near East." FAO Technical Bulletin No. 35. pp 294; Munier, P. (1973): *Le Palmier-dattier-Techniques agricoles et productions tropicales*; Maison Neuve et Larose, Paris. 217pp.

14. Manniche, *An Ancient Egyptian Herbal*, 133–134.

15. Abbiw, *Useful Plants of Ghana,* 68.

16. Ibid.

17. Manniche, *An Ancient Egyptian Herbal,* 119.

18. Grime, *Ethno-Botany of the Black Americans,* 106.

19. hooks, *Sisters of the Yam.*

20. Foster, Steven, *Men's Health and What You Need to Know About Saw Palmetto* (Eureka Springs, AZ: Steven Foster Group, 2000).

EPILOGUE

1. Hocker, Cliff, "Environmental Awareness, Blacks Measure Up Favorably," *Black Enterprise,* January 27, 2008.

2. Ibid.

3. Ibid., 20.

4. Maathai, Wangari, *The Green Belt Movement: Sharing the Approach and the Experience,* new expanded edition (New York: Lantern Books, 2004), 6.

5. Ibid., 40.

6. Ibid., 40–45.

7. Ibid., 47.

8. Ibid., 48.

9. Ibid., 6.

10. Turnbull, *The Forest People*, 260.

11. Quote provided with permission from Wadja Egnankou through the Goldman Prize

12. Nommo, Nzingha A., *African Seeds of Life* (self-published, Oak Park, IL: Jill Patrice Bunton, a.k.a. Nzinga Amma Nommo, 2002).

13. Lachance, A., "The Sweet Smell of Success," *IDRC Bulletin* 21 (2): 1–3 (2002).

14. IUPAC.org (2000).

15. Agribusiness in Sustainable Natural African Plant Products, A-SNAPP (2003).

16. African Shea Butter, www. Africansheabuttercompany.com (accessed August 29, 2003).

17. The Temple of Yehwe, Vodou Medicine, Max-G Beauvoir, www.vodou.org, seminars and workshops.

18. Central Intelligence Agency, "Grenada," in *The World Fact Book*, www.cia.gov/library/publications/the-world-factbook/print/gj.html (last updated and accessed January 8, 2008).

19. www.fao.org/docrep/v4084e/v4084eOb.htm (last accessed January 8, 2008).

20. Gullah/Geechee Sea Island Coalition, PO Box 1207, St. Helena Island SC 29920, (843) 838-1171.

4. http://library.thinkquest.org/27209/animal.htm (last accessed December 17, 2007).

5. Feeley-Harnik, *Cloth and the Creation of Ancestors in Madagascar*, 93.

GLOSSARY

1. Makinde, *African Philosophy, Culture, and Traditional Medicine*, 92.

2. Thompson, *Flash of the Spirit*, 9.

3. Feeley-Harnik, G., *Cloth and the Creation of Ancestors in Madagascar*, in *Cloth and Human Experience*, ed. Weiner, A. and J. Schneider

Glossary

Abortifacient—a substance that terminates a pregnancy

Alterative—a treatment that causes a gradual positive change in the body

Amoebicidal—destructive to amoebas

Analgesic—a substance used to relieve pain

Anaphrodisiac—a substance used to decrease libido and enhance sexual appetite, the opposite of aphrodisiac

Anesthetic—a substance that blocks sensation and dulls pain

Anthelmintic—a substance used to expel parasites (worms) from the body

Anodyne—a substance that relieves pain by lessening the sensitivity of the brain or nervous system

Antibilious—a substance that helps remove excess bile from the body

Antibiotic—an agent with biological activity that inhibits the growth of microorganisms (bacteria, fungus, etc.)

Antidiabetic—an agent used to lower glucose level in blood, used to treat diabetes

Antidiarrhea—an agent used to control and relieve diarrhea

Antiemetic—a substance used to alleviate nausea, vomiting, and headache pain

Antilithic—a substance used to prevent urinary calculi (mineral stones) or to demolish them if formed

Antiphlogistic—an anti-inflammatory agent used to treat fever and inflammation

Antipyretic—a substance used to reduce body temperature and quell fever

Antirheumatic—an agent used to alleviate rheumatism; may also be used to slow down the progression of some autoimmune diseases

Antiscorbutic—a substance used to prevent or relieve scurvy

Antiseptic—a substance used to prevent infection by hindering the growth of infectious agents

Antispasmodic—a substance that prevents or relieves spasms

Antisyphilitic—an agent used against syphilis

Antitussive—a substance used to relieve coughing

Antivenomous—an agent used to counteract venom or poison from a snake or insect bite

Antiviral—a substance used to treat viral infection

Aphrodisiac—a substance used to increase libido and sexual desire

Appetizer—an agent that stimulates the appetite

Aromatherapeutic—inhalation of fragrances (oils or herbs) having a beneficial effect on mood and health

Aromatic—having an aroma or fragrant property

Astringent—an agent that causes constriction of body tissues, decreasing the flow of blood or other fluid

Balsam—an aromatic resin produced by a tree, for example balsam of Peru and balsam of Tolu, which contain appreciable amounts of benzoic acid, cinnamic acid, or both, or their esters

Bitter—a tonic made with herbs or roots and usually blended with alcohol

Calmative—a substance with sedation properties that induces relaxation

Cardiac stimulant—a substance that promotes circulation and increases cardiac efficiency

Carminative—an antispasmodic agent used against digestive tract cramps and flatulence

Cathartic—a laxative or other agent used to purify the bowels

Cephalic—relating to the head

Cholagogue—a substance that increases the discharge of bile from the body

Cordial—a stimulant or tonic

Decongestant—an agent used to relieve congestions by reducing swelling in membranes, often used to relieve nasal congestion

Demulcent—an agent used to reduce swelling and discomfort by coating membranes with a soothing barrier

Dentifrice—a liquid, paste, or powder used to maintain proper dental hygiene

Detergent—a compound or mixture used to clean

Diaphoretic—a substance used to encourage perspiration

Digestives—agents that aid in digestion of food in the body

Disinfectant—an antimicrobial agent used to kill infectious, disease-causing organisms

Diuretic—a substance that increases the rate of urine production by the kidneys

Emetic—a substance used to induce vomiting (emesis)

Emmenagogue—a substance that encourages menstrual bleeding

Emollient—an agent that softens, moisturizes, and soothes skin

Expectorant—a substance used to loosen and expel mucus or secretions in the lungs

Febrifuge—a medicine used to decrease body temperature or fever

Galactogogue—a substance used to increase milk production

Germifuge—an agent that eliminates germs

Hemostatic—a substance or procedure used to stop bleeding

Herpectic—pertaining to or resembling herpes

Hypnotic—a substance used to induce sleep; a treatment for insomnia; anesthesia

Laxative—a substance used to encourage bowel movements and to relieve constipation

Medicinal—a substance that has the qualities of a medicine; dealing with or pertaining to the treatment of illness or injury

Mucilaginous—having a moist, sticky quality resembling mucilage; secreting mucilage

Narcotic—a substance that induces sleep

Nervine—a substance that acts upon the nerves; particularly to calm the nerves

Parasiticide—an agent used to treat or rid the body or external parasites (e.g., lice, ringworm)

Pectoral—having to do with the breast or chest

Poultice—from the Latin *porridge*, medicated mass, usually soft, wet, and warm, spread on cloth and applied to inflamed or injured area

Purgative—an agent used to cleanse or purge, especially in terms of the bowels

Refrigerant—an agent used to reduce fever

Relaxant—an agent used to relieve muscular or nervous tension

Resolvent—a substance used to reduce inflammation or swelling; also a liquid used to dissolve over substances

Rubefacient—a substance that irritates the skin causing redness and warmth

Sedative—a substance that reduces anxiety or irritability and has a tranquilizing, calming effect

Soporific—an agent that induces sleep

Stimulant—an agent that temporarily increases activity, causing a stimulating effect

Stomachic—having to do with the stomach; an agent that is beneficial to the stomach or digestion

Styptic—astringent or haemostatic; an agent that constricts tissue or blood vessels, stopping blood flow

Tonic (nutritive)—an agent that restores nutrition to the body

Tonic (systemic)—an agent that affects a particular body system, bringing energy

Vermifuge—an agent that causes the body to expel intestinal worms

Vesicant—a substance that causes blisters

Vulnerary—a substance used in the treatment and healing of wounds

CROSS-CULTURAL AFRICAN HERBAL TREATMENTS

Agbo—African infusion method (Yoruba)

Agunmu—pounded medicine (Yoruba)

Arts—dance, drumming, rattles, song sticks, praise song, performance, masks, costumes used in combination to produce healing (several African societies)

Ase—the power of spoken word and herbal medicine combined. An *onisegun* (herbalist) pulverizes tree medicine and other herbs and puts them on the tip of the tongue before uttering potent incantations.[1] (Yoruba)

Ashe—such a powerful and mysterious word that it is really untranslatable.[2] It is part spiritual command and it is very desirable during divination because it enables smoother contact with ancestors and spirits. Frequently I use this word in an herbalist's manner to describe healing elixir present in the liquid essence of a tree, plant, root, flower, bud, berry or leaf. (Yoruba)

Decoction—made by extracting medicines from tougher parts of the plant including roots, bark or berries; decoction is accomplished by simmering the tough parts of the tree in a covered pan of water over medium-low heat for thirty minutes to five hours depending on degree of toughness. Once this process is complete *ashe* is readily available for healing work in the brew, which is formally called a decoction but can be called a potion or by another name. (cross-cultural; mainly Western)

Divination—Tree medicine isn't simply harvested and worked like a biomedicine: it has a recognized metaphysical and spiritual content. As such divination plays a role in what medicine to use, how much, and for which individual. Problems can be addressed by a skilled diviner; thus it is its own healing modality in African holistic medicine.

Etu (**burnt medicine**)—slowly charring ingredients in a pot. *Etu* is consumed as is or used as body rub. (Yoruba)

Igbere—a Yoruban technique of injecting medicine in the manner of a vaccination.

Infusion—can be either water-based or oil-based. Water-based infusions are teas containing *ashe*, also called tisanes or brews. Infusions are made by extracting the volatile oils of a plant in the following manner: pour boiling distilled water over the herb and keep it covered for thirty

minutes to one hour. Heating in water for a longer time on a very low temperature on the stovetop infuses tougher herbs; the pot should be tightly covered to retain healing medicine rather than allowing it to escape into the air. (cross-cultural; mainly Western, more likely called tea or used as bath in Africa and African diaspora)

Iwa rere and *Iwa pele*—a level-headed energy; mind, body, spirit in balance; tranquility; coolness, even-handed temperament when attempting divination, conjuration, or healing. (Yoruba)

Kia—a transcendent state, which allows spirits to move through the healer, usually brought about through dance. (!Kung/South African)

Maceration—helps release the volatile oils and delicate scents of buds and flowers. To macerate buds, mash them up in a mortar with a pestle or pulse for thirty seconds in a mini food processor. (cross-cultural; started in Khemet)

Magical spirit hand—often a special hand used in the preparation and consumption of magical or spiritual medicines. This hand is typically the left hand, considered the magical hand, as many people are right-handed. (Africa and African diaspora)

Mampiboaka tromba—calling spirit directly. Through *Mampiboaka tromba* call out good or bad spirits to state the intentions behind bringing mental, physical, or metaphysical illness, identification of what type of spirit is involved, under whose agency it is working, seeing what they want, how it should be dressed, and what they require to leave. This technique may include praise songs. Once the *tromba* (royal ancestor spirit) says its name it is no longer considered powerful.[3] (Malagasy/Sakalava people)

Mafutas—a practice using fat, with or without trees and herbs, from a wide variety of animals, reptiles, and insects including bull, baboon, eagle, puff adder, porcupine, monkey, wildebeest, iguana, hippopotamus, giraffe, and chameleon for medicinal value. The animal is selected for magical, spiritual, and mythological significance as well as for the vitamins/minerals/enzymes it contains.[4] (Zulu/South Africa)

Oil-based infusion—extraction of the volatile oils from herbs by soaking the herbs in oil. (started in Khemet, now used in Americas and elsewhere)

Olugbohun—an amulet with special *ase* prepared in the horn of a bull and partially wrapped in symbolic cloth.[5] (Yoruba)

Oruka—medicinal (herbal) ring; medicine that is worn externally to affect the holistic health of the patient. (Yoruba)

Patience—It should go without saying, but many feel it's OK to forcefully handle tree medicines, yet in the process they lose the potentiality of the plant to heal. Patience is critical. (cross-cultural)

Praise—As you have learned, each tree has a protocol for planting, growing, harvesting, and using. Even though you may be uninitiated, it is vital to be thankful to the tree for giving its life force in an effort to assist your healing work. (African diaspora)

Prayer—Generally thanksgiving is given at time of planting, during the growing process, at harvest, and when processing tree medicines. This can take the form of a chant, praise song, or prayer that incorporates your faith. (cross-cultural)

Tincture—extraction of healing medicines from herbs created by using 100-proof alcohols such as vodka, grain alcohol, or rum. The concentrations of volatile oils are greater in tinctures than through infusion or decoction. (cross-cultural, especially New World)

Toddy—Since the ancient African civilizations at Axum, Kush, Nubia, Khemet, and Egypt, African healers have combined herbal infusions with wine or other alcoholic beverages. (cross-cultural, today mostly Jamaica)

Bibliography

Abbiw, D. K. *Useful Plants of Ghana: West African Uses of Wild and Cultivated Plants*. London: Intermediate Technology Publications and the Royal Botanic Gardens KEW, 1995.

Abrahams, R. D. *African American Folktales: Stories from Black Traditions in the New World*. New York: Pantheon Books, 1999.

———. *African Folktales*. New York: Pantheon Books, 1983.

Alldridge, T. J. *The Sherbro and Its Hinterland*. London: MacMillan and Co., 1901.

Amen, R. U. N. *Metu Neter Vol. 1: The Great Oracle of Tehuti and the Egyptian System of Spiral Cultivation*. New York: Kamit Publications, 1990.

Anderson, Martha G., and Christine Mullen Kreamer. *Wild Spirits Strong Medicine: African Art and the Wilderness*. New York: Center for African Art, 1989.

Barham, H. *Hortus Americanus Particular of the Island of Jamaica*. Kingston: A. Aikman, 1725.

Baring, A., and J. Cashford. *The Myth of the Goddess: Evolution of an Image*. New York: Penguin Books, 1993.

Barrett, L. *The Sun and the Drum: African Roots in Jamaican Folk Tradition*. Kingston: Sangster's (in association with Heinemann), 1976.

Bernard, I. "Time, Space, and the Evolution of Afro-American Society on British Mainland North America." *American Historical Review* 85, no. 1: 1980–1968.

Biesele, M. "Folklore and Ritual of Kung Hunter-Gatherers" (doctoral dissertation). Cambridge, MA: Harvard University, 1975.

Bird, S. R. *Sticks, Stone, Roots and Bones: Hoodoo, Mojo & Conjuring with Herbs*. St. Paul, MN: Llewellyn Worldwide, 2004.

———. *Four Seasons of Mojo: An Herbal Guide to Natural Living.* St. Paul, MN: Llewellyn Worldwide, 2006.

Blao, H. "Producing Essential Oils in West Africa." *IDRC Bulletin*, 2003.

Boughman, A. L., and L. O. Oxendine. *Herbal Remedies of the Lumbee Indians.* Jefferson, NC, and London: McFarland and Company, 2003.

Boulos, L. *Medical Plants of North America.* Algonac, MI: Reference Publications, Inc., 1983.

Breadfruit Institute, National Tropical Botanical Garden, 2007. www.ntbg.org/breadfruit/uses (last accessed January 4, 2008).

Bremness, L. *The Complete Book of Herbs.* New York: Viking Studio Books, Penguin Putnam, 1994.

———. *Fragrant Herbal: Enhancing Your Life with Aromatic Herbs and Essential Oils,* New York: Little, Brown and Company, 1998.

Brown, D. J. "Pomegranate Juice Improves Carotid Artery Health and Lowers Blood Pressure in Patients with Carotid Artery Stenosis" (clinical update). *Herbal Gram: The Journal of the American Botanical Council*, issue 65, 2005: 28–30.

Buckley, A. D. *Yoruba Medicine.* Brooklyn, NY: Athelia Henrietta Press, Inc. Publishing in the Name of Orunmila, 1997.

Caldecott, M. *Myths of the Sacred Trees.* Rochester, VT: Destiny Books, 1993.

Camino, L. A. "The Cultural Epidemiology of Spiritual Heart Trouble." *Herbal and Magical Medicine: Traditional Healing Today*, eds. James Kirkland, Holly F. Mathews, C. W. Sullivan III, and Karen Baldwin. Durham, NC, and London: Duke University Press, 1997.

Carawan, G., and C. Carawan, eds. *Ain't You Got a Right to the Tree of Life? The People of Johns Island, South Carolina—Their Faces, Their Words, Their Songs.* Athens, GA: University of Georgia Press, 1994.

Carper, Jean. *Food: Your Miracle Drug: Preventing and Curing Common Health Problems the Natural Way.* New York: Harper Collins, 1993.

Cassidy, F. G., and R. B. Le Page. *Dictionary of Jamaican English.* Cambridge, U.K.: Cambridge University Press, 1967.

Copney, C. V. *Jamaican Culture and International Folklore, Superstitions, Beliefs, Dreams, Proverbs, and Remedies.* Raleigh, NC: Pentland Press, 1999.

Courlander, H. *A Treasury of Afro-American Folklore.* New York: Marlowe & Co., 1996.

Cumber Dance, D., ed. *From My People: 400 Years of African American Folklore.* New York: W. W. Norton & Company, 2002.

Davidson, B. *The Lost Cities of Africa.* Boston: Little, Brown and Company, 1959.

Diallo, Y., and M. Hall. *The Healing Drum: African Wisdom Teachings.* Rochester, VT: Destiny Books, 1989.

Doumbia, A., and N. Doumbia, PhD. *The Way of the Elders: West African Spirituality and Tradition.* St. Paul, MN: Llewellyn Worldwide, 2004.

Drewal, H. J. "Arts and Divination Among the Yoruba: Design and Myth." *African Journal* 14. nos. 2–3, 1987.

Duke, J. A. *Herbs of the Bible: 2000 Years of Plant Medicine.* Loveland, CO: Interweave Press, 1990.

Edwards, V. H. *The Aromatherapy Companion: Medicinal Uses/Ayurvedic Healing/Body-Care Blends/Perfumes and Scents/Emotional Health and Well-Being.* North Adams, MA: Storey Books, 1999.

Emerick, A. S. J. *Jamaica Duppies.* Woodstock, MD: 1916.

Fett, S. *Working Cures: Healing, Health and Power on Southern Slave Plantations.* Chapel Hill & London: University of North Carolina Press, 2002.

Fontenot, W. L. *Secret Doctors: Ethnomedicine of African Americans.* Westport, CT, and London: Bergin & Garvey, 1994.

Glassman, S. A. *Vodou Visions.* New York: Villard Books, 2000.

Goodwine, M. *The Legacy of Ibo Landing: Gullah Roots of African American Culture.* Atlanta: Clarity Press, 1998.

Grime, W. E. *Ethno-Botany of the Black Americans.* Algonac, MI: Reference Publications, 1979.

Guerry, V. *Life with the Baoule.* trans. Nora Hodges; Washington, DC: Three Continents Press, 1975.

Hamilton, V. *The People Could Fly: American Black Folktales.* New York: Alfred P. Knopf, 1985.

Harris, J. B. *Iron Pots and Wooden Spoons.* New York: Ballantine Books, 1989.

Harsch, E. "Making Trade Work for Poor Women." *African Recovery.* 2001.

"Herbs, Spices and Flavorings." http://en.wikipedia.org/wiki/Allspice (last modified January 8, 2008; last accessed January 8, 2008).

Hocker, C. "Environmental Awareness, Blacks Measure Up Favorably." *Black Enterprise.* January 27, 2008.

Hohman, J. G. *Pow-Wows or Long-Lost Friend: A Collection of Mysterious and Invaluable Arts and Remedies.* Pomeroy, WA: Health Research Publishers, 1820.

hooks, b. *Sisters of the Yam: Black Women and Self-Discovery.* Cambridge: South End Press, 1993.

Houghton, P., et al (1994). "Activity of Extracts of *Kigelia Pinnata* Against Melanoma and Renal Carcinoma Cell Lines." *Planta Medica* 60 (5): 430–433.

Huttman, T., ed. *The Africa News Cookbook: African Cooking for Western Kitchens.* New York and London: Penguin Books and Africa News Service, 1985.

Hyatt, H. M. *Folklore of Adams County, Illinois: Memoirs of the Alma Egan Hyatt Foundation.* New York: The E. Cabella-French Printing and Publishing Corporation, 1935.

Illes, J. *Earth Mother Magic: Ancient Spells for Modern Belles.* Gloucester, MA: Fairwinds Press, 2001.

Jeffries. "The Image of Woman in African Cave Art," *Journal of African Civilizations,* 6:1 (1988).

Jones, J. H. *Bad Blood: The Tuskegee Syphilis Experiment—A Tragedy of Race and Medicine.* New York: The Free Press, 1981.

Joseph, J. A., PhD, A. Underwood, and D. A. Nadeau, M.D. *Color Code: A Revolutionary Eating Plan for Optimum Health.* New York: The Philip Lief Group, Inc. 2002.

Karade, B. I., and J. D. Baldwin. "Pre-Historic Nations." *The Handbook of Yoruba Religious Concepts,* ed. L. Olumide. York Beach: Weiser Books, 1994.

Katz, R. *Boiling Energy: Community Healing Among the Kalahari Kun.* Cambridge, President and Fellows of Harvard College, 1982.

Khan, M., and S. Mlungwana. "Short Report: y-Sitosterol, a Cytotoxic Sterol from Markhamia Zanzibarica and Kigelia Africana." *Fitoterapia* 70 (1999): 96–97.

Labouret, H. *La Divination par le Souris a la Côte d'Ivoire.* Bulletin du Musee d'Ethnographie du Trocadero 8, 1935.

LaGamma, A. (essay by Pemberton, J.). *Art and Oracle: Spirit Voices of Africa.* New York: The Metropolitan Museum of Art, 2000.

Lancashire, R. J. University of West Indies, Department of Chemistry, Kingston 7, Jamaica c. 1994 (updated and accessed August 4, 2003).

Lappe, F. M., and A. Lappe. *Hope's Edge: The Next Diet for a Small Planet.* New York: Jeremy P. Tarcher, Penguin Group, 2002.

Latz, P. *Bushfires and Bushtucker: Aboriginal Plant Use in Central Australia.* Alice Springs, NT, Australia: IAD Press, 1995.

Little, K. L. *The Mende of Sierra Leone.* London: Routledge and Kegan Paul, 1951.

Maathai, W. *The Greenbelt Movement* (revised edition). New York: Lantern Books, 2003.

Mack, C., and D. Mack. *A Field Guide to Demons, Fairies, Fallen Angels, and Other Subversive Spirits.* New York: Henry Holt, 1998.

Makinde, M. A. *African Philosophy, Culture and Traditional Medicine.* Athens, OH: Ohio University Center for International Studies, Africa Series Number 53, 1988.

"Mali." *Funk & Wagnalls New Encyclopedia.* 2006. A WRC Media Company. http://www.worldalmanac.com (last accessed Jauary 20, 2008).

Manniche, L. *An Ancient Egyptian Herbal.* Great Britain: British Museum Press and the University of Texas Press, 1989.

McClusky, P. *Art from Africa: Long Steps Never Broke a Back.* Princeton, NJ; Seattle, WA: Princeton University Press and Seattle Art Museum Press, 2002.

McCormick, J. "The Vegetation of the New Jersey Pine Barrens" in the anthology *Pine Barrens: Ecosystem and Landscape,* ed. Richard T. T. Forman, New Brunswick and London: Rutgers University Press, 1979: 229–244.

McIntyre, A. *The Complete Woman's Herbal: A Manual of Healing Herbs and Nutrition for Personal Well Being and Family Care.* New York: Henry Holt Books, 1994.

McNair, J. *Squash Cookbook.* San Francisco: Chronicle Books, 1989.

Mitchell, F. *Hoodoo Medicine.* Columbia, SC: Summerhouse Press, 1999.

Montet, P. *Phoenix: Eternal Egypt.* Phoenix Press, 2000.

Morton, J. "Breadfruit." *Fruits of Warm Climates.* Miami, FL: Julia F. Morton, 1987, 50–58. http://www.hort.purdue.edu/newcrop/morton/breadfruit.html (accessed January 5, 2008).

———. "Orange." *Fruits of Warm Climates.* Miami, FL: Julia F. Morton, 1987, 134–143. www.hort.purdue.edu/newcrop/morton/orange.html (last accessed January 18, 2008).

———. "Pomegranate." *Fruits of Warm Climates.* Miami, FL: Julia F. Morton, 1987, 352–355. www.hort.purdue.edu/newcrop/morton/pomegrante.html (last accessed January 18, 2008).

Musgrave, T., and W. Musgrave. *An Empire of Plants: People and Plants That Changed the World.* London: Cassell and Co., 2000.

Mutwa, V. C. *Zulu Shaman: Dreams, Prophecies, and Mysteries.* ed. Stephen Larsen. Rochester, VT: Destiny Books, 1996.

Nickens, T. E. *Saving Spirit Trees.* Washington, DC: American Forests, 2007. www.americanforests.org (last accessed January 1, 2008).

Nommo, N. A. *African Seeds of Life.* Self-published. Oak Park, IL. Jill Patrice Bunton, a.k.a. Nzinga Amma Nommo, 2002.

Offodile, B. *The Orphan Girl and Other Stories: West African Folktales.* Northampton, MA: Interlink Publishing Group, 2001.

Olumide, L., and B. I. Karade. *The Handbook of Yoruba Religious Concepts.* San Francisco, CA: Weiser, 1994.

Omoleya, M. *Certificate History of Nigeria.* London & Lagos: Longman Group, 1986.

Onyefulu, I. *Ebele's Favorite: A Book of African Games.* London: Frances Lincoln Press, 2000.

Palmer, E. *The South African Herbal.* Cape Town, South Africa: Tafelberg Publishers Ltd., 1985.

Paravisini-Gebert, E., and M. Fernandez Olmos. *Creole Religions of the Caribbean: An Introduction from Vodou and Santeria to Obeah and Espiritismo.* New York: New York University Press, 2003.

———. *Sacred Possessions: Voodoo, Santeria, Obeah and the Caribbean.* New Brunswick, NJ, March 1997.

Payne-Jackson, A., and M. C. Alleyne. *Jamaican Folk Medicine: A Source of Healing.* Kingston, Jamaica: University of West Indies Press, 2004.

Perkins, L. "Duppy Plants in Jamaica." *Jamaica Journal* 3 (1):17–21.

Pinto, A. C. de Q., M. C. R. Cordeiro, S. R. M. de Andrade, F. R. Ferreira, H. A. de C. Filgueiras, R. E. Alves, and D. E. Kinpara. "Annona Species" International Centre of Underutilized Crops, Southampton, UK, 2005.

Puckett, Newbell Niles. *Folk Beliefs of the Southern Negro.* Montclair, NJ: Patterson Smith, 1968.

Purchon, Nerys. *Handbook of Natural Healing.* St. Leonards, NSW: Allen & Unwin, 1998.

Rashidi, R. "African Goddesses" in *Civilizations* 6:1. New Brunswick & London: Transaction Publishers, 2002.

Reading International Solidarity Center. www.risc.org.uk/bogolan/index.htm (last accessed December 17, 2007).

Redd, D. "Hatsheput," in *Black Women in Antiquity.* New Brunswick & London: Transaction Publishers, 2002.

Roodt, V. "Kigelia Africa." *The Shell Field Guide to the Common Trees of the Okavango Delta and Moremi Game Reserve. Gaborone.* Botswana: Shell Oil Botswana, 1992.

Roy, C. *Art of the Upper Volta Rivers.* Meudon, France: Alain and Francoise Chaffin, 1987.

"Sausage Trees at Phyto Trade Africa." www.phtotradeafrica.com/products/sausage.htm (accessed December 21, 2007).

Scheub, H. *A Dictionary of African Mythology: The Mythmaker as Storyteller.* Oxford: Oxford University Press, 2000.

Schildkrout, E., and C. A. Keim. *African Reflections* (exhibition catalog). New York: American Museum of Natural History, 1990.

Scott, G. *Headwraps: A Global Journey.* Cambridge, MA: Perseus Books and New York: Public Affairs Books, 2003.

Simpson, G. E. "Folk Medicine in Trinidad." *Journal of American Folklore* 75 (1962): 298.

———. *Black Religions in the New World.* New York: Columbia University Press, 1978: 115.

Sloane, Sir H. A. *Voyage to the Islands, Madera, Barbados, Nieves, St. Christopher's and Jamaica.* London: British Museum, 1725: 2, 61.

Smith, A. C. "Angiosperm Evolution and the Relationship of the Floras of Africa and America," in Meggers, B. J., E. S. Ayensu, and W. D. Duckworth (eds.), *Tropical Forest Ecosystems in Africa and South America: A Review.* Washington, DC: Smithsonian Institution (1973), 49–61.

Snow, L. F. *Walkin' Over Medicine.* Boulder, San Francisco, Oxford: Westview Press, 1993.

Some, M. P. *The Healing Wisdom of Africa: Finding Life Purpose Through Nature, Ritual and Community,* New York: Jeremy P. Tarcher/Putnum, 1999.

Stoller, P., and C. Olkes. *In Sorcery's Shadow.* Chicago & London: University of Chicago Press, 1987.

Studley, V. *The Art and Craft of Handmade Paper.* Mineola, NY: Dover Publications, 1990.

Susie, D. A. *In the Way of Our Grandmothers: A Cultural View of Twentieth-Century Midwifery in Florida.* Athens and London: University of Georgia Press, 1988.

Taylor, J. Y. "Talking Back: Research as an Act of Resistance and Healing for African American Women Survivors of Intimate Male Partner Violence," in *Women and Therapy* vol. 25, no. 34. Hawthorn Press Inc., 2002.

Thompson, R. F. *Black Gods and Kings* (exhibition catalog). Los Angeles: UCLA Flower Museum of Cultural History, 1976.

———. *"Babalawo."* Alawode Ifayemi, informant to R. F. Thompson, 71.

———. *Flash of the Spirit: African and Afro-American Art and Philosophy.* New York: Vintage Books, 1987.

Trudge, C. *The Tree: A Natural History of What Trees Are, How They Live and Why They Matter.* New York: Crown Publishers, 2006.

Turnbull, C. *The Forest People: A Study of the Pygmies of the Congo.* New York: Touchstone/Simon & Schuster, 1962.

Turner, L. D. *Africanisms in the Gullah Dialect.* Arno Press and New York Times, 1969.

Umeh, J. A. *After God Is Dibla: Igbo Cosmology, Divination and Sacred Science in Nigeria,* vol. 2, London: Karnak House, 1999.

Van Sertima, I., ed. *Black Women in Antiquity.* Piscataway, NJ: Transaction Publishers, 2002.

Van Wyk, B., and N. Gericke. *People's Plants—A Guide to Useful Plants of Southern Africa.* Briza Publications, Pretoria, 2000.

Voeks. R. A. *Sacred Leaves of Candomblé: African Magic, Medicine, and Religion in Brazil.* Austin, TX: University of Texas Press, 1997.

Walker, Barbara. *The Woman's Encyclopedia of Myths and Secrets.* Edison, NJ: Castle Books, 1991.

Wedenoja, W. *Religion and Adaptation in Rural Jamaica* (doctoral dissertation). University of California, San Diego, 1978: 81.

Weenen, H., et al. "Anti-Malarial Activity of Tanzanian Medicinal Plants." *Planta Medica* 56 (1990): 368–370.

Weil, A. *Spontaneous Healing: How to Discover and Enhance Your Body's Natural Ability to Maintain and Heal Itself.* New York: Ballantine Books and Fawcett Columbine, 1995.

Williams, L., and C. S. Finch. "The Great Queens of Ethiopia" in *Civilizations* 6:1. New Brunswick & London: Transaction Publishers, 2002.

Worwood, Dr. V. A. *The Complete Book of Essential Oils and Aromatherapy,* Novato, CA: New World Library, 1991.

————. *The Fragrant Heavens: The Spiritual Dimension of Fragrance and Aromatherapy.* Novato, CA: New World Library, 1999.

Yarbrough, C. *Journal of African Civilizations*, ed. Ivan Van Sertima, 2002.

————. "Female Style and Beauty in Ancient Africa," in *Civilizations* 6:1. New Brunswick & London: Transaction Publishers, 2002.

Zaslavsky, Claudia. *Africa Counts: Number and Pattern in African Cultures*, third ed. Chicago: Lawrence Hill Books, 1999.

Zone10.com. http://www.zone10.com/tech/NASA/ Fyh.htm, Plants for Clean Air Council (accessed April 23, 2008).

www.ghana.co.uk/history/fashion/adrinka_adinka symblos.htm (last accessed December 17, 2007).

Index